PHARMACOLOGY - RESEARCH, SAFETY TESTING AND REGULATION

AMOXICILLIN

MEDICAL USES, MECHANISM OF ACTION AND POTENTIAL ADVERSE EFFECTS

WYATT A. LEARY
AND
LOGAN M. KRUSE
EDITORS

New York

For permission to use material from this book please contact us:
Telephone 631-231-7269; Fax 631-231-8175
Web Site: http://www.novapublishers.com

Additional color graphics may be available in the e-book version of this book.

Library of Congress Cataloging-in-Publication Data

ISBN: 978-1-62948-489-1

Library of Congress Control Number: 2013952267

Published by Nova Science Publishers, Inc. † New York

Contents

Preface

Amoxicillin represents the lead substance of the aminopenicillin group of beta-lactames, which is characterized by a broader antibacterial spectrum and acid-stability compared to penicillin G. In this book, the authors present current research in the study of the medical uses, mechanisms of action and potential adverse effects of amoxicillin. Topics discussed include microfibers of biodegradable polymers loaded with amoxicillin; the occurrence, fate and effects of amoxicillin in aquatic systems; accurate instrumental analytical methods for the quality control of amoxicillin in the pharmaceutical industry; and the pharmaceutical properties and clinical applications of amoxicillin.

Chapter I – The chapter deals with the fabrication, structural aspects, chemical-physical characteristics, in vitro release and antibacterial properties of mats of non-woven fibers of poly (ε-caprolactone) (PCL), poly (lactic acid) (PLA) and blends of poly (lactic acid) and poly (ε-caprolactone) loaded with different amounts of Amoxicillin antibiotic (AMOX) using electrospinning technique. Amoxicillin drug was used alone or intercalated in layered double hydroxide (LDH) nanoparticles by co-precipitation method and then successfully encapsulated at different concentrations into PCL, PLA and blends of PLA and PCL. The nano-fibrous structure of all mats was composed of individual, uniform and randomly oriented fibers. The addition of AMOX and LDH/AMOX at different concentrations caused only slightly increasing of the average diameter and the presence of rare beads on the surface of the microfibers. For all electrospun samples the release curves present a sustained release behavior, although an initial rapid drug release was found. The initial high-rate drug release period was followed by a second step in which the release is slow, extending for long time. The comparison of the release curves showed that the release of amoxicillin protected into the clay is slower that the release of the drug alone. Different release kinetics of the two polymers (PCL and PLA) were found. Comparing the release amount with that predicted by the mixture rule a preferential incorporation of amoxicillin into poly(lactic acid) can be inferred. The properties of the loaded membranes and their capability for local delivery of antibiotics make them suitable for biomedical applications.

Chapter II – Antibiotics have been widely used for some decades. Although these substances are developed to perform a biological effect, little attention has been given to the presence of these pharmaceuticals in the environment, namely in aquatic systems. For instance, frequent use of veterinary antibiotics raise concerns related to direct contamination of water and increase in antibiotic resistance of microorganisms. In the aquatic environment, antibiotics can be dissolved in the water and might affect non-target organisms due to bioaccumulation and biomagnification processes. One group of antibiotics largely used to treat infections caused by susceptible bacteria is the penicillins. The present work addresses an up-to-date review on the occurrence, fate and effects of amoxicillin, the most used antibiotic within the β-lactams class, in aquatic systems. It brings up important questions, regarding the uncertainties related to the behavior of amoxicillin in aquatic systems as well as the risks associated with its occurrence.

Chapter III – New fast, robust, and accurate instrumental analytical methods for the quality control of the widely-used active pharmaceutical ingredient amoxicillin are of high importance for the pharmaceutical industry. This chapter summarizes recent published new approaches and methods for qualitative and quantitative analysis of amoxicillin and refers to the analysis of other beta-lactam antibiotics. Its main focus is on separation techniques such as high performance liquid chromatography (HPLC) and capillary electrophoresis (CE) and on spectroscopic methods like mid-infrared- (MIR), near-infrared- (NIRS), terahertz- and Raman-spectroscopy. Other focuses are chemiluminescence and UV-vis spectrometric methods, electrochemical methods and paper analytical devices.

Chapter IV – Amoxicillin represents the lead substance of the aminopenicillin group of beta-lactams, which is characterized by a broader antibacterial spectrum and acid-stability compared to penicillin G. It is the hydroxylated derivative of ampicillin and is used orally because of its nearly full oral bioavailability and its high tissue diffusion, however, it has a short terminal half-life of only 1 - 1.5 hours. Amoxicillin is a very popular antibiotic, especially by family practitioners. In 2010, amoxicillin was the fifth most commonly prescribed generic medication of the USA. Like for all other beta-lactams its bactericidal activity is based on the inhibition of the bacterial cell wall synthesis by inactivating enzymes, so-called penicillin binding proteins, which are located in the cell membrane. Amoxicillin is active against a broad spectrum of Gram-positive (not *S. aureus*, not *E. faecium*) and Gram-negative (not *P. aeruginosa*, *Enterobacter spp.*, *Klebsiella spp.* etc.) bacteria, however, it has no activity against anaerobic bacteria. In the last decades the emergence and spread of β-lactamases has become a major problem for the medical use of Amoxicillin. The β-lactamases - including plasmid-mediated AmpC enzymes, extended-spectrum β-lactamases (ESBL) and carbapenemases – mediate resistance to different or all classes of beta-lactams. Nevertheless, the medical use of amoxicillin still is various. Especially in infections of the ENT area it is commonly used and well proven for the empiric treatment of otitis media, sinusitis, tonsillitis, and pharyngitis. However, it is also indicated for non-severe respiratory infections such as community-acquired pneumonia as well as for uncomplicated urinary tract infections in woman. Furthermore, oral amoxicillin administration is recommended by national and international guidelines for prophylaxis of infective endocarditis, especially for the treatment of infective endocarditis due to enterococci or oral streptococci. Amoxicillin is generally considered a well-tolerated drug; however, there are several potential adverse effects and contraindications the physician has to take in mind. The most important contraindication is a known allergy or hypersensitivity against penicillin's or any other beta-lactams. The administration of amoxicillin to a patient with a history of beta-lactam hypersensitivity can lead to severe anaphylactic reactions which sometimes can be fatal. Other adverse events are occurrence of gastrointestinal symptoms, such as diarrhoea, or exanthema (on average 8%). Especially in patients with infectious mononucleosis, other viral diseases, or lymphocytic leukemia exanthema is significantly more frequent.

In: Amoxicillin ISBN: 978-1-62948-489-1
Editors: W. A. Leary and L. M. Kruse © 2014 Nova Science Publishers, Inc.

Chapter I

Microfibers of Biodegradable Polymers Loaded with Amoxicillin

Eduardo Valarezo[1,2,*], *Loredana Tammaro*[1], *Luis Cartuche*[2], *Miguel Meneses*[3], *Chabaco Armijos*[2], *Silvia González*[2], *Omar Malagón*[2] and *Vittoria Vittoria*[1]

[1]Dipartimento di Ingegneria Industriale, Universitàdegli Studi di Salerno, Fisciano (SA), Italy

[2]Departamento de Química, Universidad Técnica Particular de Loja, Loja, Ecuador

[3]Departamento de Ciencias Agropecuarias y de Alimentos, Universidad Técnica Particular de Loja, Loja, Ecuador

Abstract

The chapter deals with the fabrication, structural aspects, chemical-physical characteristics, in vitro release and antibacterial properties of mats of non-woven fibers of poly (ε-caprolactone) (PCL), poly (lactic acid) (PLA) and blends of poly (lactic acid) and poly (ε-caprolactone)

[*] Tel: +593 7 2570 275, ext. 2512. E-mail: bevalarezo@utpl.edu.ec.

loaded with different amounts of Amoxicillin antibiotic (AMOX) using electrospinning technique.

Amoxicillin drug was used alone or intercalated in layered double hydroxide (LDH) nanoparticles by co-precipitation method and then successfully encapsulated at different concentrations into PCL, PLA and blends of PLA and PCL. The nano-fibrous structure of all mats was composed of individual, uniform and randomly oriented fibers. The addition of AMOX and LDH/AMOX at different concentrations caused only slightly increasing of the average diameter and the presence of rare beads on the surface of the microfibers. For all electrospun samples the release curves present a sustained release behavior, although an initial rapid drug release was found. The initial high-rate drug release period was followed by a second step in which the release is slow, extending for long time. The comparison of the release curves showed that the release of amoxicillin protected into the clay is slower that the release of the drug alone. Different release kinetics of the two polymers (PCL and PLA) were found. Comparing the release amount with that predicted by the mixture rule a preferential incorporation of amoxicillin into poly(lactic acid) can be inferred. The properties of the loaded membranes and their capability for local delivery of antibiotics make them suitable for biomedical applications.

Keywords: Amoxicillin, Electrospinning, Nanofibers, Poly(e-caprolactone), Poly (lactic acid)

Introduction

Electrospinning is a versatile technique for preparing nano and microfibers of natural and synthetic polymers [1]. The accumulation of these non-woven or aligned fibers produces the so called fibrous mats [2], fibrous fabrics [3] or fibrous membranes [4]. Through this process it is possible to produce polymer or polymer composite fibrous mats with high surface to volume ratio [5]. The solution properties, such as viscosity, concentration, surface tension and electrical conductivity as well as processing parameters, such as voltage, type of collector, solution flow rate, needle diameter and needle-collector distance can influence the properties and the morphology of the electrospun fibers [6, 7]. Solution properties and processing parameters can be optimized according to the final required characteristics [8]. The electrospun nanofibers were found to have wide applications in several fields such as filtration [9], wound healing

[10], protective clothing [11], drug delivery [12] and biomedical areas [13, 14] such as scaffold for tissue engineering [15, 16].

Poly(ε-caprolactone) (PCL) is a semi-crystalline biodegradable polyester with a glass transition temperature of about −60°C and a low melting point of around 60°C, which could be a handicap in some applications. Therefore, PCL is generally blended [17] or modified (e.g., copolymerisation, crosslink [18]). This synthetic polymer is currently used in a number of biomedical applications due to its mechanical properties, miscibility with a large range of other polymers, biocompatibility [19], biodegradability, good drug permeability and slow biodegradability [20].

Polylactic acid or polylactide (PLA) is a thermoplastic aliphatic polyester derived from renewable resources, such as corn starch (in the United States), tapioca roots, chips or starch (mostly in Asia), or sugarcane (in the rest of the world). It can biodegrade under certain conditions, such as the presence of oxygen and without the presence of oxygen. This is a biodegradable polymer with different biomedical applications because of its mechanical properties and biocompatibility [19].

Amoxicillin (AMOX) is a bacteriolitic, β-lactam antibiotic used to treat bacterial infections caused by susceptible microorganisms, one of the most common antibiotic for children [21, 22]. Recently, a study on mice indicated successful delivery using intraperitoneally injected amoxicillin-bearing microparticles, showing a growing interest in the controlled delivery of this drug. AMOX is used to treat infections caused by bacteria in ear, lung, nose, urinary tract and skin infections. It is also used before surgery to prevent infections [21].

The incorporation of low molecular weight active molecules into polymer matrices has the disadvantage that the migration and the release of the molecule cannot be easily predicted and controlled. To face these problems we have recently proposed a method for fixing active molecules (antiinflammatory, antibiotic, and antimicrobial) into an inorganic compound able to hold them, allowing a very slow and controlled release in selected conditions [23-25]. In particular, layered double hydroxide (LDHs), or hydrotalcite like compounds, have been considered as active molecule delivery vehicles, because of their anion exchange properties [26]. These compounds, also known as "anionic clays" have the general formula $[M(II)_{(1-x)}M(III)_x(OH)_2](A_{x/n})\ mH_2O$ where M(II) is a divalent cation such as Mg, Ni, Zn, Cu or Co and M(III) is a trivalent cation such as Al, Cr, Fe or Ga, A^{n-} an anion of charge n such as CO_3^{2-}, Cl^-, NO_3^- or organic anions [27-33]. Modified LDHs can be prepared with simple procedures, at high level of purity. They are cheap and eco-compatible and can be organically modified with a variety of organic anions, generally much more numerous than organic cations, commonly involved in the modification of cationic clays (i.e. fillosilicates). This latter characteristic will make these layered compounds a very attractive class of lamellar solids because the release of active molecules in molecule-intercalated layered materials is potentially controllable.

In this chapter we present the preparation of fibrous composites by using electrospinning technique, obtained by encapsulating an antibiotic drug, amoxicillin and LDH-amoxicillin nano-hybrids into biodegradable PCL, PLA and PLA/PCL. The structure, morphology and thermal behavior of the electrospun fibers were analyzed, and correlated to the pristine polymer properties. The release of the active AMOX was studied in physiological solution and showed interesting effects, regarding the different concentrations.

Materials and Methods of Investigation

Materials

Poly(ε-caprolactone) (PCL, M_n=80000 Da), $Zn(NO_3)_2*6H_2O$, $Al(NO_3)_3*9H_2O$, Acetone and Amoxicillin (AMOX) (potency ≥900 μg mg^{-1}) were purchased from Sigma-Aldrich, Poly-(lactic acid) (PLA) (containing about 4.0 mol % of D-lactoyl units) was purchased in pellet form from Nature Works® Co., and used as received without further purification.The nano-hybrid LDH-amoxicillin anion was prepared by coprecipitation method according to a reported procedure (Frunza et al., 2008). Intercalation of amoxicillin into ZnAl-LDH can be tuned by varying the Zn/Al ratio because the amount of anion depends on the excess of positive charge in the clay, in turn depending on the Zn/Al ratio. This ratio can generally assume values between 2 and 4, according to the reaction conditions. We tried to reach the maximum of positive charge, with the following procedure: 20 mL of an aqueous solution of $Zn(NO_3)_2*6H_2O$ (2.5 g, 8.4 mmol) and $Al(NO_3)_3*9H_2O$ (1.6 g, 4.3 mmol) were added to 20 mL of aqueous solution of amoxicillin sodium (0.9 g, 2.3 mmol) in a conical flask under stirring and under nitrogen flow. After about 4 hours the pH slowly reaches the value of 7.5 by dropwise addition of 1M aqueous NaOH solution. The precipitate was washed several times with decarbonated distilled water and dried at 50°C for 24h in vacuum oven.

Elemental analysis indicated that we obtained an intercalated nano-hybrid with formula:

$$[Zn_{0.65}Al_{0.35}(OH)_2](C_{16}H_{18}N_3O_5S)_{0.35}\cdot 1.2\ H_2O$$

In this formula the amoxicillin content is 54 wt% of the total nano-hybrid weight. Of course by varying the Zn/Al ratio we can vary the amount of anion amoxicillin and, in turn, its percentage. The size mean dimension of the powders was measured as 1.2 micron.

Methods

Preparation of Electrospun Membranes

Electrospinning of PLA, PCL, PLA/PCL mixtures, their AMOX filled solutions and PCL/LDH-AMOX composites were carried out at room temperature using solutions in acetone (polymer percentage 17.5% wt/wt). The voltage was varied between 20 and 30 kV (HV Power Supply, Gamma High Voltage Research, Ormond, FL).

A copper wire was mounted in the spinneret having an inner diameter of 0.8 mm and used as the positive electrode. Grounded aluminium foil was used as the counter electrode and mounted at different distance (20-30 cm) from the spinneret. Continuous polymer, polymer mixtures and composite polymer mixtures were collected on the aluminium foil in fibrous mat form. Electrospinning conditions were optimized to produce fibrous mats with bead-less fibers (so called bead-on-string).

Differential Scanning Calorimetry (DSC)

DSC measurements were carried out using a Mettler DSC 822/400 thermal analyzer instrument having sub-ambient capability. About 2-3 mg sample was placed in an aluminium pan and heated at a rate of 10°C/min from 0 to 250°C in a nitrogen atmosphere.

Thermogravimetric Analysis (TGA)

Thermoanalytical characterizations were performed by a Mettler TC-10 thermobalance operating at 5°C/min heating rate, under air flow, from 25 to 800°C. Degradation temperature (T_d) is reported as the midpoint of the degradation step.

X-ray Diffraction (XRD)

XRD data were collected using an automatic Brukerdiffractometer (equipped with a continuous scan attachment and a proportional counter), with the nickel filtered Cu Kα radiation (λ = 1.54050 Å) and operating at 40 kV and 40 mA. The diffraction scans were recorded at 2θ = 2-40, step scan 0.03 of 2θ and 3s of counting time.

Scanning Electron Microscopy (SEM)

The morphology and the diameter of the electrospun nanofibers were analysed by a scanning electron microscope (SEM Mod. LEO 420, Assing, Italy). All samples were sputter coated with gold (Agar Automatic Sputter Coater Mod.B7341, Stansted, UK) at 40 mA for 180 s prior the analysis. The fibers diameter distribution was determined by Sigma ScanPro 5. About 500 fibers were considered, taking their dimensions respect to the reference bar of SEM image.

Ultraviolet Spectroscopy (UV-VIS)

The in vitro study of amoxicillin release was performed by measuring the absorbance at 228 nm using an ultraviolet spectrophotometer (model UV-2401, SHIMADZU). The tests were performed using rectangular specimen of 25 cm^2 placed into 25 mL of physiological saline solution, stirred at room temperature and 100 rpm in an orbital shaker (VDRL MOD. 711+, AsalS.r.l.). The release medium was withdrawn at fixed time intervals and replenished with fresh medium.

Antibacterial Activities In Vitro

The inhibitory activity of the electrospun nanofibers charged with different concentrations of AMOX was evaluated by the disc diffusion method according to the specifications of the document M2-A9 from the Clinical and Laboratory Standards Institute [34]. A criogenic (-80°C) reserve of each strain was used to make the overnight broth culture. An aliquot of the criogenic reserve of *S. aureus* and *E. coli* was inoculated in two 7 ml Tryptic soy broth tubes while *E. faecalis* was inoculated in 7 ml BHI broth. Each bacteria was adjusted to 0.5 McFarland in 0.9% sodium chloride solution previous to the inoculation in MHA plates. Three membranes in shape of disc of 6 mm diameter were placed onto MHA plates. The procedure was repeated three times per bacteria. The plates were inverted face down and incubated at 35°C for 24 hours.

AMOX work solution (1mg/mL) was used as positive control [35], three 6 mm diameter wells were made in three MHA plates, one per strain, 25 μl of the AMOX work solution was injected in each well. The activity against the same three bacteria was evaluated using the agar well diffusion method as described by Boyanova et al. [36] and Kroiss et al. [37]. As negative control, five 6 mm diameter discs of nanofibers without AMOX were sterily placed onto one MHA plate and incubated under the same conditions above. All data were statistical analyzed by means of Student's t-test with α 0,05.

Results

Morphology and Structure

Many internal as well as external parameters can influence the electrospinning process and, as a consequence, the fiber morphology. Indeed it is difficult to isolate the effect of each parameter since they all are interrelated. For this reason, typically a trial-and-error approach has been employed by varying the solution properties and the spinning parameters until uniform defect-free fibers are obtained.

Table 1 summarizes the percentages of PLA/PCL/AMOX/LDH-AMOX used, the optimal electrospinning conditions applied and the average diameter of the fibers for all samples prepared.

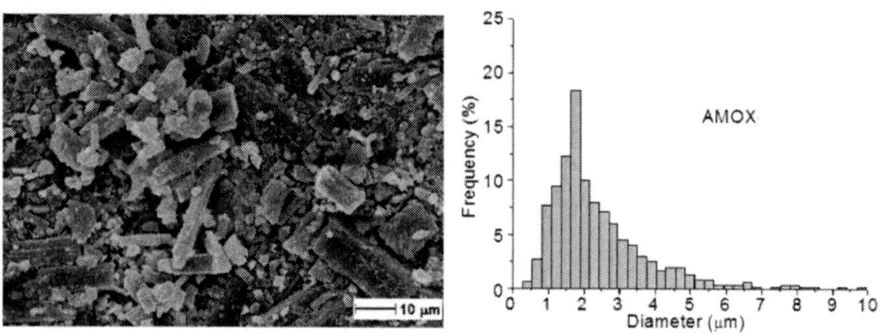

Figure 1. SEM micrographs and crystal dimension of pristine amoxicillin. [38]

Table 1. Composition (PLA/PCL/AMOX/LDH-AMOX), processing parameters and average diameter values of fibers fabricated by electrospinning (flow rate: 4 mL/h. SD: standard deviation, diameter values are means of 500 determinations)

Sample	PLA (wt%)	PCL (wt%)	AMOX (wt%)	LDH/ AMOX (wt%)	Distance (cm)	Voltage (kV)	Fiber Diameter (μm)	SD (μm)
AMOX	-	-	100	-	-	-	2.37	1.41
PCL	-	100	-	-	30	30	1.01	0.50
PCL-A3	-	100	3	-	30	30	1,17	0.71
PCL-A5	-	100	5	-	30	30	1.31	0.77
PCL-A7	-	100	7	-	30	30	1.40	0.88
LDH/ AMOX	-	-	54	100	30	30	1.23	0.81
PCL-LDH/ AMOX3	-	100	1.62	3	30	30	1.64	1.01
PCL-LDH/ AMOX5	-	100	2.70	5	30	30	1.66	1.35
PCL-LDH/ AMOX7	-	100	3.78	7	30	30	1.78	1.43
PLA	100	-	-	-	20	20	2.52	0.53
PLA-A3	100	-	3	-	20	20	2.58	0.49
PLA-A5	100	-	5	-	20	20	2.66	1.17
PLA-A7	100	-	7	-	20	20	3.22	0.99
P75	75	25	-	-	25	20	2.43	0.48
P75-A3	75	25	3	-	25	20	2.53	0.77
P75-A5	75	25	5	-	25	20	2.60	1.23
P75-A7	75	25	7	-	25	20	2.63	1.68
P50	50	25	-	-	25	20	1.98	0.51
P50-A3	50	50	3	-	25	20	2.04	0.86
P50-A5	50	50	5	-	25	20	2.10	1.23

Sample	PLA (wt%)	PCL (wt%)	AMOX (wt%)	LDH/ AMOX (wt%)	Distance (cm)	Voltage (kV)	Fiber Diameter (μm)	SD (μm)
P50-A7	50	50	7	-	25	20	2.30	1.24
P25	25	75	-	-	25	25	1.51	0.46
P25-A3	25	75	3	-	25	25	1.97	0.72
P25-A5	25	75	5	-	25	25	2.05	1.09
P25-A7	25	75	7	-	25	25	2.22	1.10

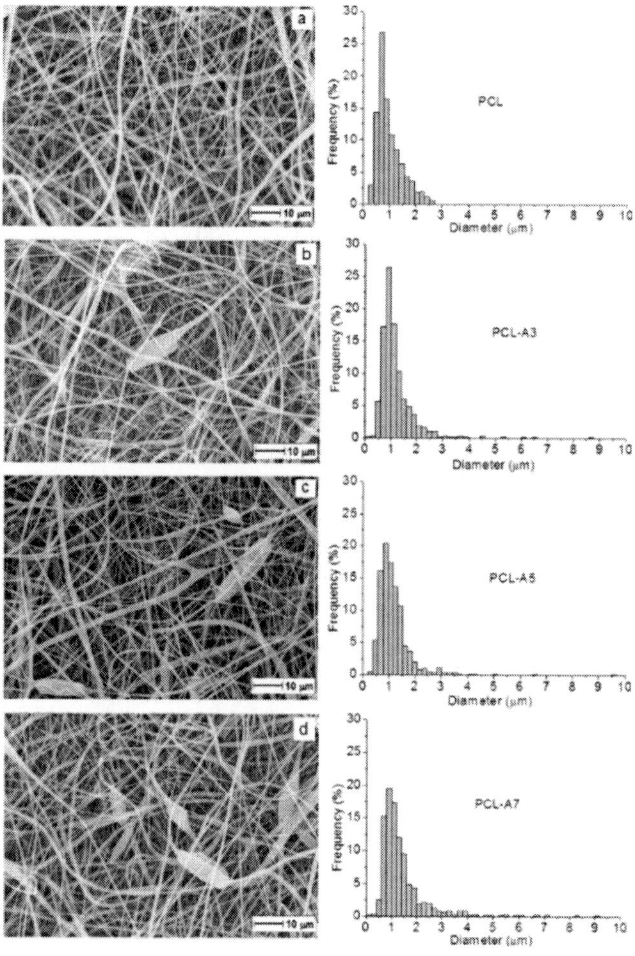

Figure 2. SEM micrographs and diameter distribution of PCL (a), PCL-A3 (b), PCL-A5 (c), PCL-A7 (d). [38].

In Figure 1 [38] a SEM micrograph of pristine amoxicillin and the crystal dimension distribution are shown. Pure amoxicillin is a highly crystalline material with a flat rod shape of dimensions ranging between 1 and 3 μm and centred at about 2 μm.

The SEM micrographs and the diameter distribution of the obtained fibrous membranes of PCL and PCL loaded with amoxicillin (PCL-A3, PCL-A5, PCL-A7) are show in Figure 2 [38]. The nanofibrous structure of pristine PCL sample is characterized by individual, uniform, and randomly oriented fibers with an average diameter ranging around 0.8 μm. The addition of amoxicillin did not give rise to evident change in the morphology of the sample.

Some rare beads appear, possibly due to clusters of the AMOX molecules on the surface of the microfibers.

The addition of the amoxicillin drug, intercalated in a layered double hydroxide, (LDH/AMOX) at different concentrations caused no noticeable change in the morphology of the PCL based membranes. Moreover it resulted in electrospun fibers with a very similar or slightly higher average diameter around 0.8–1.2 μm, in comparison with pure PCL, although a prevailing number of fibers with higher dimensions is observable. Some rare beads appear (Figure 3c and d) [39], possibly due to clusters of the nano-hybrid on the surface of the microfibers.

Blends of poly(lactic acid) (PLA) and poly(ε-caprolactone) (PCL), loaded with different amounts of Amoxicillin antibiotic were electrospun too.

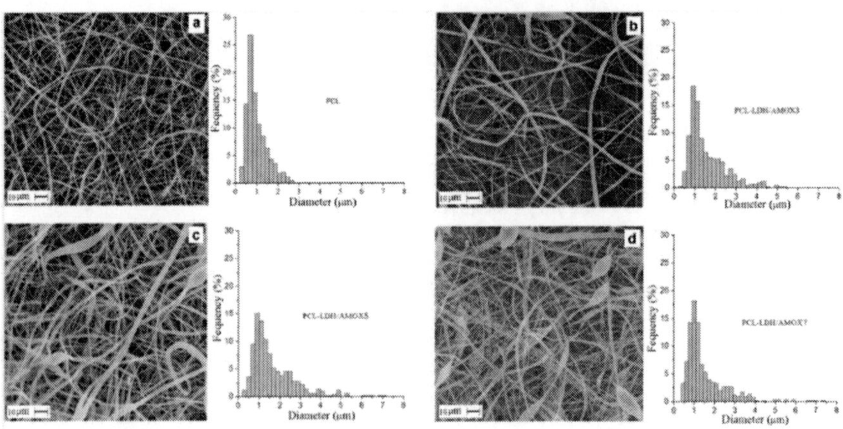

Figure. 3. SEM micrographs of PCL (a), PCL-LDH/AMOX3 (b), PCL-LDH/AMOX5 (c) and PCL-LDH/AMOX7 (d). Reprinted from Applied Clay Science, 72, Valarezo, E. et. al., 104-109, 2012 [39], with permission from Elsevier.

Lower distance and lower voltage (20 cm and 20 KV) than those used for the formation of PCL fibers (30 cm and 30 KV) are required for PLA fiber formation. Increasing the amount of PCL in the mixture, higher voltage and higher distance were needed for the formation of polymer mixture fibers. The average diameter of PCL fibers was 1.01 μm. This value increased with increasing the amount of PLA: 1.51 μm for P25 (25wt% PLA, 75 wt% PCL), 1.98 μm for P50 (50 wt% PLA, 50 wt% PCL), 2.43 μm for P75 (75 wt% PLA, 25 wt% PCL) and 2.52 μm for PLA. The average diameter increases also with increasing the amount of AMOX in the composites fibers. Since the AMOX is insoluble in acetone, it is incorporated into the fibers as crystal particles with unchanged dimension. The presence of large AMOX crystals into the fibers (Figure 4) contributes to increase the average diameter.

The X-ray diffractograms were performed to investigate the crystalline structure of the membranes. Figure 5 [38] reports the diffraction patterns of AMOX powders, pure PCL and PCL-AMOX fibers. The AMOX powders are very crystalline (Figure 5a), showing the most intense X-ray reflections at 12.1, 15.1, 18.1 and 19.4 of 2θ. The pristine electrospun PCL and all the filled samples show the crystalline structure of PCL well developed with the main diffraction peaks appearing at 21.4 and 23.8 of 2θ. Interestingly, observing the diffractograms of the filled PCL it can be noticed that even in the sample with the higher concentration of AMOX (PCL-A7) the crystalline diffraction patterns of AMOX do not appear at all. Probably the AMOX, encapsulated into the PCL fibers, is not allowed to crystallize and exists as amorphous molecular aggregates or solid solution into the fibers.

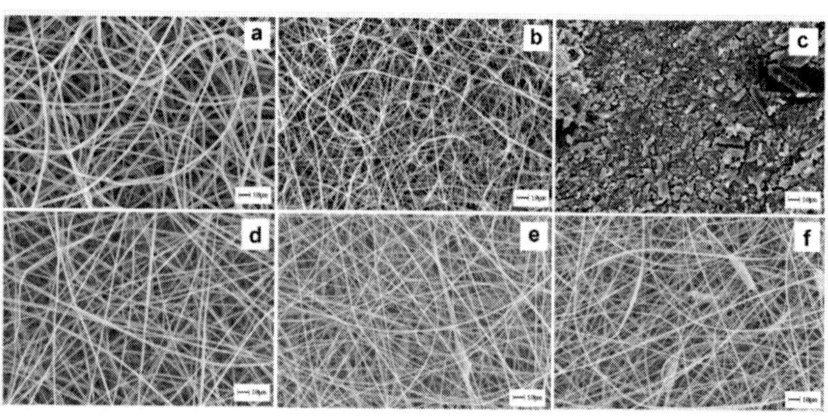

Figure 4. SEM micrographs of selected samples: PLA (a), PCL (b), AMOX (c), P50 (d), P50-A5 (e) and P50-A7 (f).

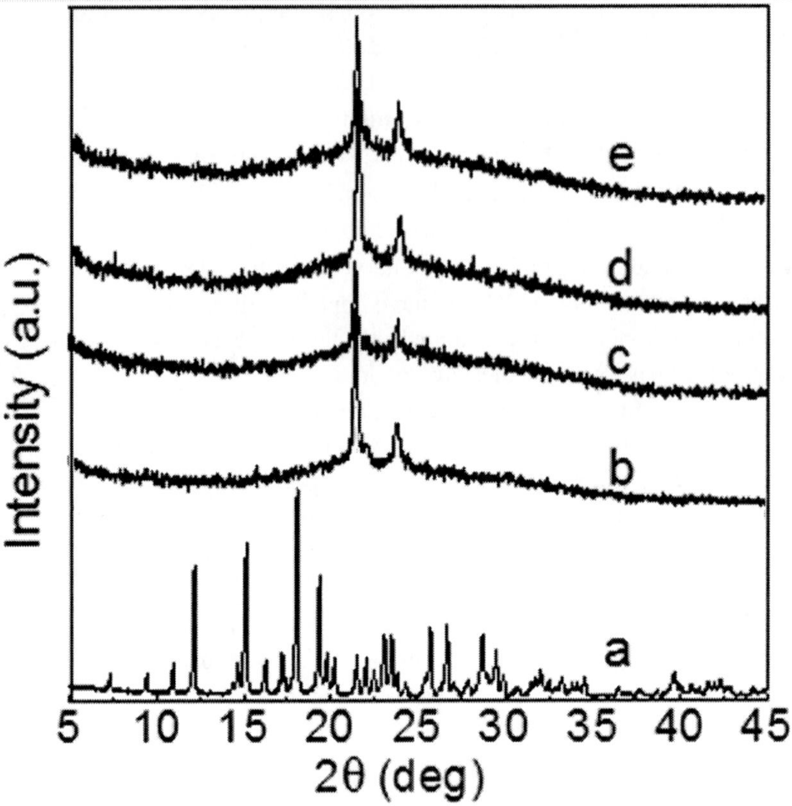

Figure 5. XRD diffractograms of pure AMOX (a), PCL (b), PCL-A3 (c), PCL-A5 (d), and PCL-A7 (e). [38]

This result has been already found by other authors and is confirmed by the thermal properties.

As shown in Figure 6 [39] the structural order of the crystalline AMOX is lost when the anions are intercalated into the LDH lamellae. The nano-hybrid indeed (Figure 6b) shows only a reflection corresponding to the basal diffraction reflection of the hydrotalcite lamellae, appearing at 3.8 of 2θ. It corresponds to an interlayer distance of 23.2 Å, much larger than the distance when inorganic anions are intercalated, for example 7.55 Å in the case of carbonate anions. The X-ray reflections are broad indicating very small and imperfect crystals of hydrotalcite with AMOX anions intercalated in the lamellae. When the nano-hybrids are incorporated into the PCL matrix (Figure 6d, e, and f) a residual and almost undistinguishable "bump" appears at $2\theta \leq 5$ corresponding to the signal of the pristine LDH/AMOX sample.

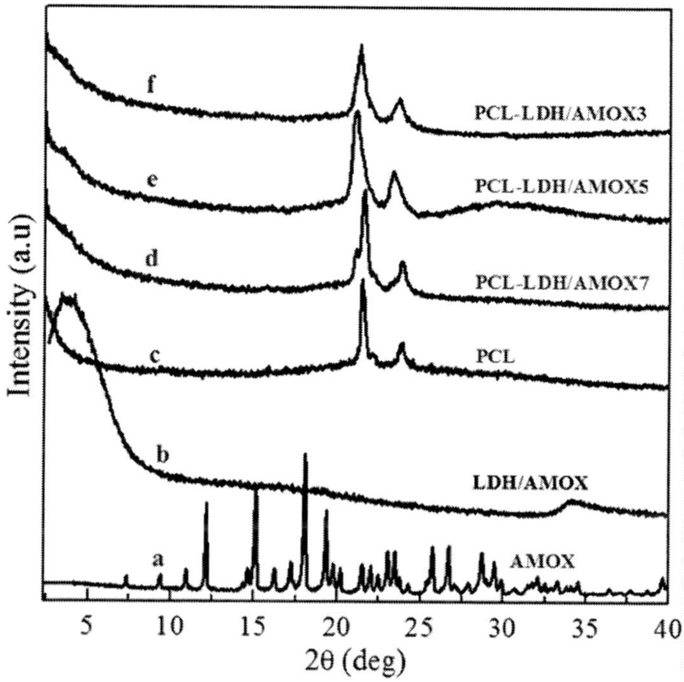

Figure 6. XRD diffractograms of AMOX (a), LDH/AMOX (b), PCL (c), PCL-LDH/AMOX7 (d), PCL-LDH/AMOX5 (e) and PCL-LDH/AMOX3 (f). Reprinted from Applied Clay Science, 72, Valarezo, E. et. al., 104-109, 2012 [39], with permission from Elsevier.

This result indicates that the nano-hybrid has lost its basal periodicity into the PCL fibers and is well dispersed inside.

A number of eight samples were chosen from the total set of electrospun blend fibers to investigate the crystallinity which would highlight the interaction between the filler and the polymer matrix. The XRD patterns of polymer mixture fibers containing PCL and PLA, composite mixture containing AMOX particles, original AMOX particles, the neat PCL and PLA fibers are shown in Figure 7. The broad pattern of the non-woven membrane (Figure 7b) can be attributed to the reflection of amorphous PLA, indicating that the evaporation of the solvent during electrospinning process is very rapid not allowing the polymer crystallization. The presence of a broad pattern in all polymeric mixture and in all composite spectra demonstrates that the PLA polymer has an amorphous structure, on which the incorporation of PCL and AMOX filler, regardless of their concentration, does not induce relevant changes.

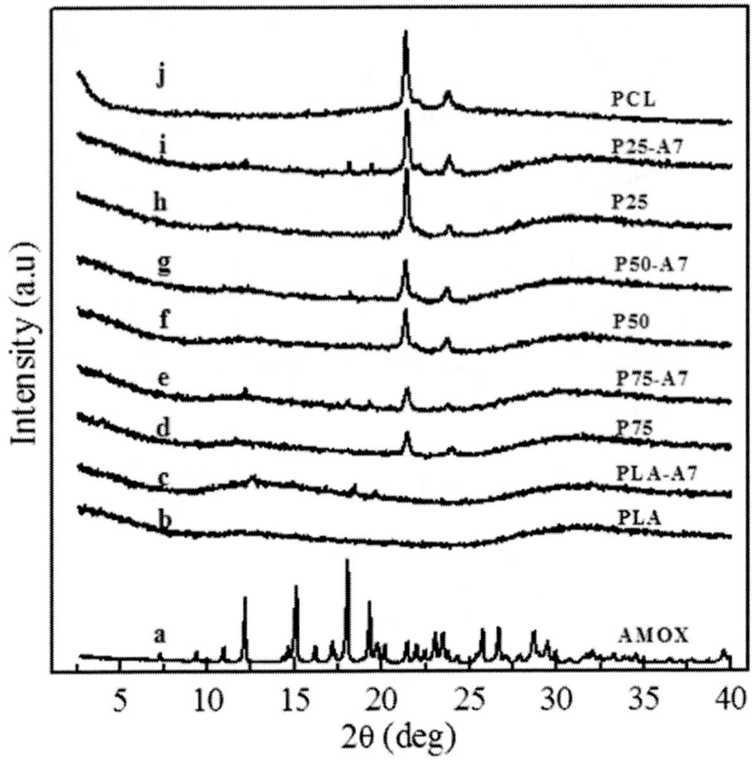

Figure 7. XRD diffractograms of pure AMOX (a), PLA (b), PLA-A7 (c), P75 (d), P75-A7 (e), P50 (f), P50-A7(g), P25 (h), P25-A7(i) and PCL (j).

For the polymer mixtures the PCL reflection intensity increases with increasing the PCL content (Figures 7c, 7e, 7g). The fibers composite containing AMOX particles show the main peaks at 12.1, 15.1, 18.1 and 19.4 of 2θ all corresponded to the structure of AMOX particles (Figure 7a) with low intensity due to the amorphous PLA phase that overlaps the filler diffraction, apart from the diffraction peaks of PCL (Figures 7d, 7f, 7h). Polymer mixtures and composite fibers resulted as physical mixtures of the constituent components.

Thermal Properties

The thermal properties are commonly studied by performing Differential Scanning Calorimetry (DSC) and Thermogravimetric Analysis (TGA). The

DSC of AMOX exhibits the first endothermic peak between 60 and 120°C with a maximum at 104°C (ΔH=347.0 J/g), which corresponds to the dehydration of AMOX.

Pure PCL shows the melting temperature (*Tm*)at about 60°C (Figure 8b) with a melting enthalpy (*ΔHm*) of 75.58 J/g. The melting curves of the filled membranes are very similar to pristine PCL, with the melting peak at about the same temperature and a lower melting enthalpy. No peak of AMOX melting is apparent, even at the highest concentration of 7%. This is further evidence that AMOX does not crystallize into the PCL membranes. The thermal parameters evaluated by DSC and TGA are reported in Table 2. These results show that the increase of the amount of AMOX in the semi-crystalline PCL nanofibers caused a reduction in the crystallinity degree (*Xc*).

As shown in Figure 9 [39] the PCL melting peak slightly shifted to lower temperatures in all PCL-LDH/AMOX composites and the melting enthalpy slightly decreased.

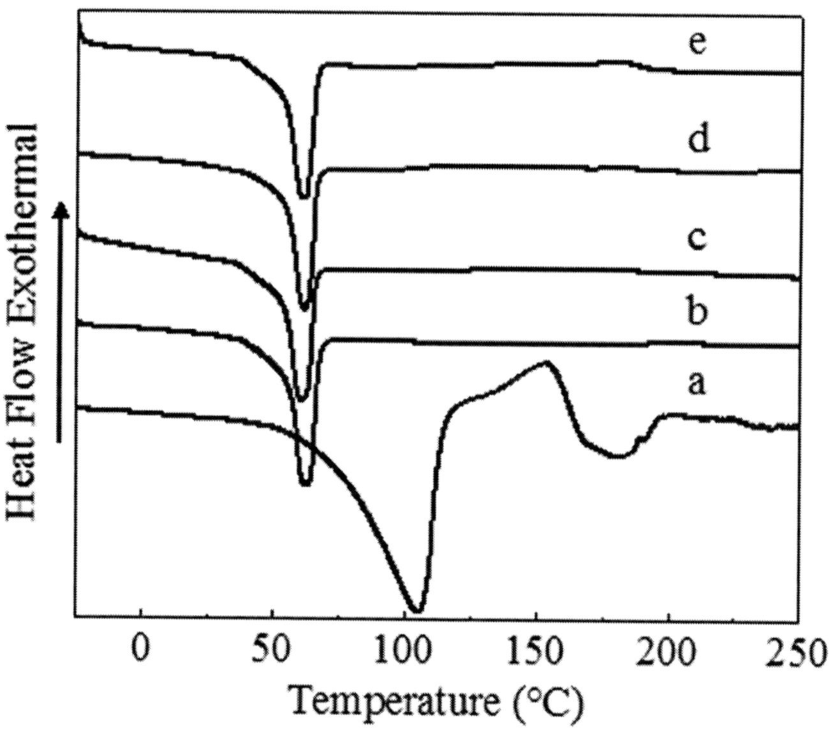

Figure 8. Differential Scanning Calorimetry (DSC) curves of pure AMOX (a), PCL (b), PCL-A3 (c), PCL-A5 (d) and PCL-A7 (e).

Table 2. Thermal parameters of electrospun fibers (AMOX: T_m = 104°C, Midpoint temperature = 306°C)

	PCL		PLA				
Sample	T_{m1} (°C)	ΔH_{m1} (J/g)	T_c (°C)	ΔH_c (J/g)	T_{m2} (°C)	ΔH_{m2} (J/g)	Midpoint temperature (°C)
PCL	63	76	-	-	-	-	385
PCL-A3	62	69	-	-	-	-	386
PCL-A5	62	69	-	-	-	-	387
PCL-A7	61	68	-	-	-	-	388
LDH/AMOX	81	76	-	-	-	-	337
PCL-LDH/ AMOX3	62	70	-	-	-	-	329
PCL-LDH/ AMOX5	61	69	-	-	-	-	325
PCL-LDH/ AMOX7	61	69	-	-	-	-	323
PLA	-	-	105	17	148	25	340
PLA-A3	-	-	103	25	148	24	344
PLA-A5	-	-	103	27	147	21	345
PLA-A7	-	-	102	29	147	19	346
P75	58	20	94	12	149	18	345
P75-A3	58	19	90	13	149	16	346
P75-A5	58	17	90	17	148	15	346
P75-A7	58	13	90	21	148	15	347
P50	58	47	89	6	150	13	350
P50-A3	58	40	89	6	150	12	350
P50-A5	58	38	89	7	150	12	353
P50-A7	58	35	88	9	150	11	354
P25	58	71	-	-	150	8	365
P25-A3	58	70	-	-	149	6	370
P25-A5	58	68	-	-	149	5	371
P25-A7	58	65	-	-	149	4	376

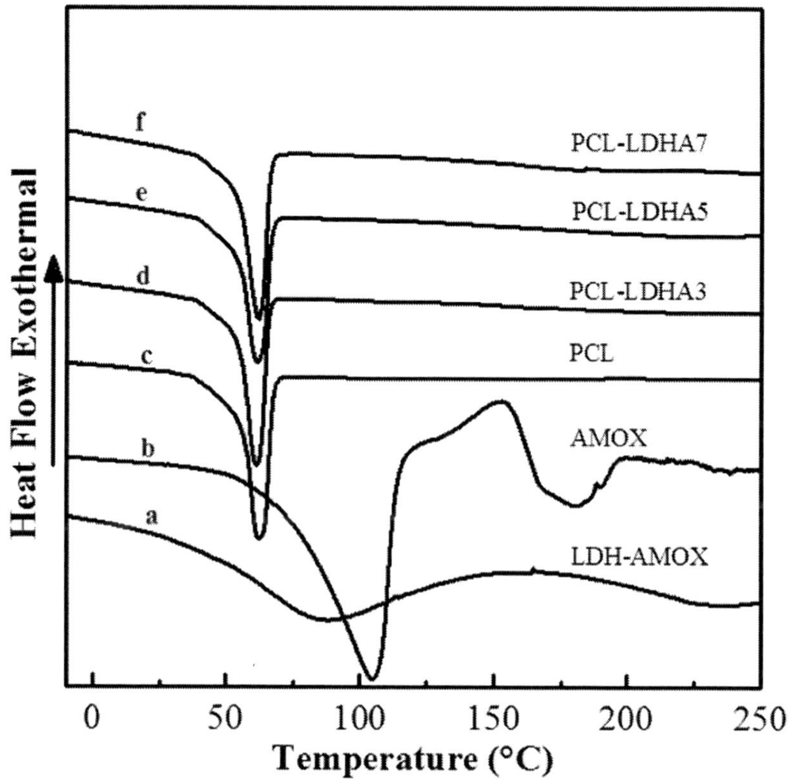

Figure 9. Differential scanning calorimetry curves of LDH/AMOX (a), AMOX (b), PCL (c), PCL-LDH/AMOX3 (d), PCL-LDH/AMOX5 (e) and PCL-LDH/AMOX7 (f). Reprinted from Applied Clay Science, 72, Valarezo, E. et. al., 104-109, 2012 [39], with permission from Elsevier.

The crystallinity (*Xc*) of the composites is slightly lower than the *Xc* value of PCL alone. The different amount of LDH/AMOX in the composites does not produce a further relevant decrease in the melting peak (*Tm*), melting enthalpy (ΔHm), crystallinity (*Xc*) and degradation temperature (Table 4).

Heating traces of representative blend samples are shown in Figure 10. The DSC curves of the electrospun samples containing both polymers show a clear endothermic peak (30-70°C) which is associated with the melting of the polycaprolactone crystalline phase and a broad exothermic peak (90-120°C) indicative of the cold crystallization of polylactide, together with the corresponding melting peak (147-150°C).

Polycaprolactone melting enthalpy (ΔH_{m1}) was sometimes difficult to calculate accurately due to the overlap with polylactide enthalpy relaxation.

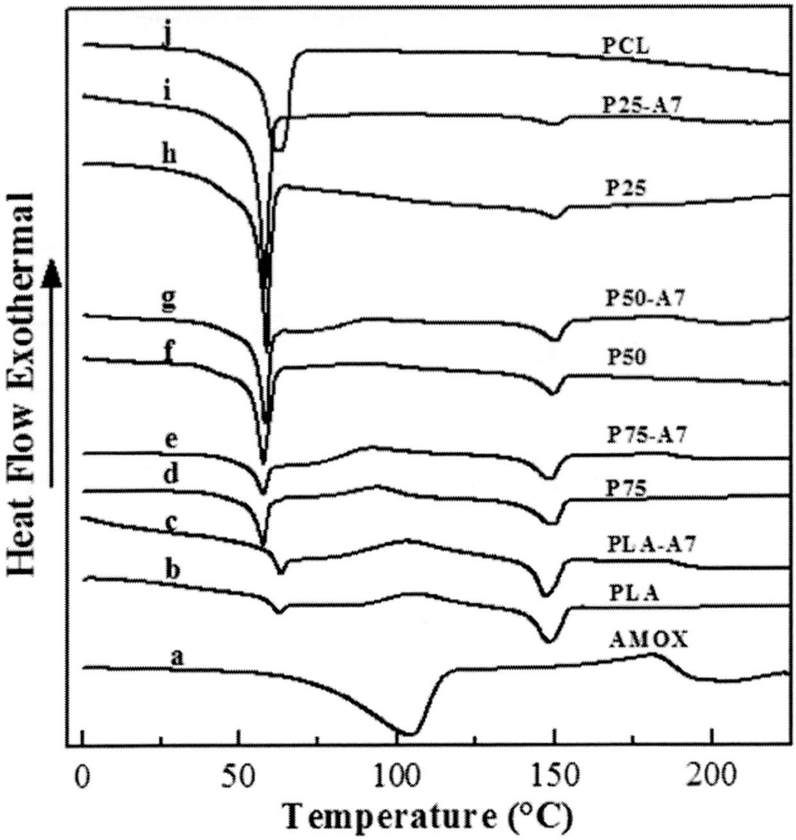

Figure 10. Differential Scanning Calorimetry (DSC) curves of pure AMOX (a), PLA (b), PLA-A7 (c), P75 (d), P75-A7 (e), P50 (f), P50-A7(g), P25 (h), P25-A7(i) and PCL (j).

As a consequence, the melting peakwas overestimated. The PCL melting peak slightly shifted to lower temperatures in all samples and the meltingenthalpy decreased when samples were loaded with AMOX. This allows inferring that thedrug was well mixed into the polymeric phase. For a given series (i.e. AMOX loaded and unloaded samples) the melting enthalpy of PCL tended to decrease with decreasing its percentage. In fact, as shown in Table 2, the ΔH_{m1}value of 76 J/g decreases up to 20 J/g in the sample with the lower PCL content (P75). The melting enthalpy of PLA also tended to decrease with its percentage. In the composites polymer mixtures no AMOX melting peak is apparent, even at the highest concentration.This is evidence that AMOX does not crystallize into the PCL membranes.

All the samples were analyzed by thermogravimetric analysis to determine the degradation temperature and confirm the content of the inorganic component in the nanohybrid materials after the thermal decomposition of the organic part in air up to 800°C. In Figure 11 [38] the thermogravimetric curves of AMOX powders, pristine PCL electrospun membrane and the filled membranes are shown. The AMOX thermogram exhibits a first step of weight loss (about 10%) that corresponding to the dehydration of AMOX. Then, AMOX is thermally decomposed at several stages whit a total weight loss of about 90%, leaving a residual mass at 800°C of about 10%. PCL thermally degrades to volatile products above 300°C and ends above 500°C. It appears that the introduction of even big amounts (7 wt%) of AMOX does not change the thermal stability of the filled samples, that show midpoint temperatures very similar to that of PCL (Table 2). This is an evidence of a good interaction between PCL and the AMOX molecules.

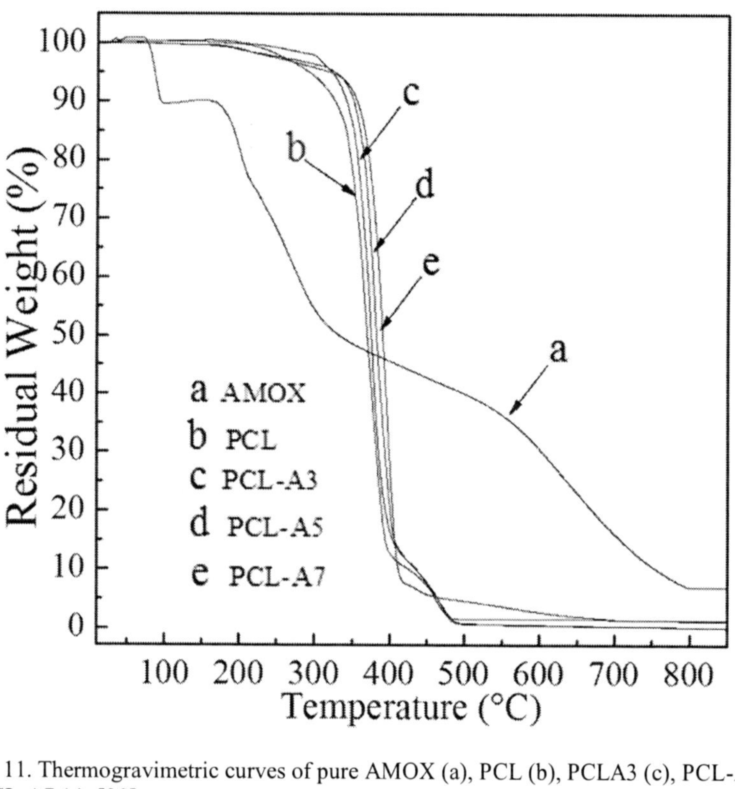

Figure 11. Thermogravimetric curves of pure AMOX (a), PCL (b), PCLA3 (c), PCL-A5 (d) and PCL-A7 (e). [38]

As shown in Figure 12 [39], LDH/AMOX undergoes the oxidative thermal decomposition in several mass loss steps: the first one, at about 85°C, was attributed to the loss of 5% of interlayer and adsorbed water molecules. The second mass loss stage between 90 and 290°C was due to dehydroxylation of the layers; the third stage was due to the oxidative decomposition of amoxicillin anion leaving a residual mass of 53% at 800°C. Interestingly the degradation of the AMOX anions intercalated into LDH lamellae (Figure 12b) is postponed, indicating a protection of the drug due to the encapsulation between the inorganic lamellae. This result has been already shown in many cases of intercalated organic molecules and results as one of the reasons for intercalating drugs into the inorganic lamellae. From the residual content at high temperature (>400°C) the inorganic content in the three filled membranes was confirmed.

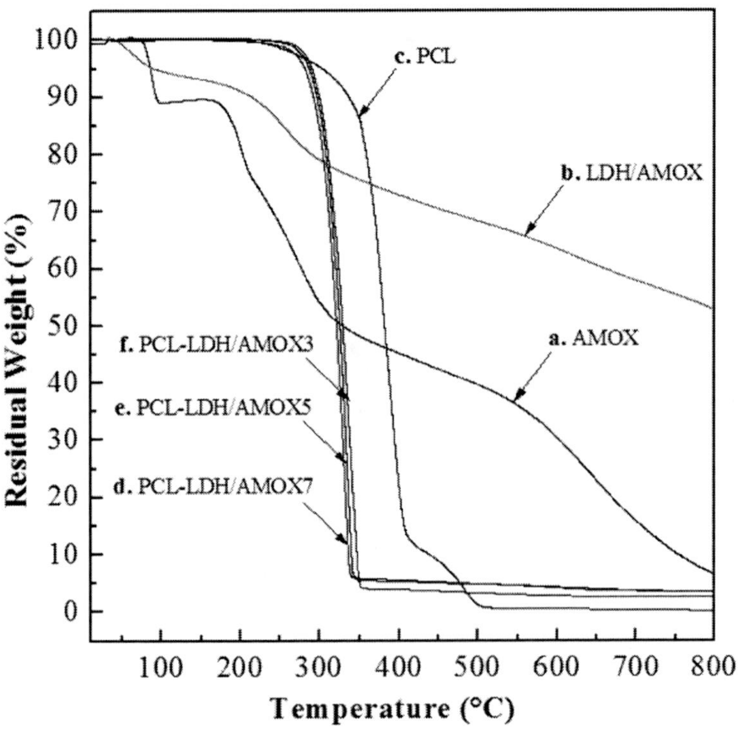

Figure 12. Thermogravimetric curves of AMOX (a), LDH/AMOX (b), PCL (c), PCL-LDH/AMOX7 (d), PCL-LDH/AMOX5 (e) and PCL-LDH/AMOX7 (f). Reprinted from Applied Clay Science, 72, Valarezo, E. et. al., 104-109, 2012 [39], with permission from Elsevier.

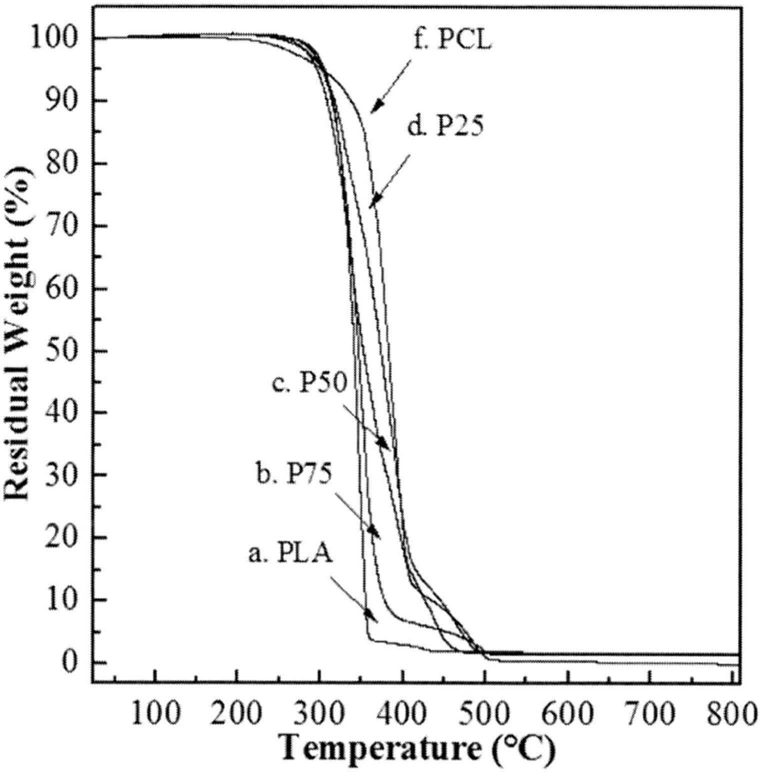

Figure 13. Thermogravimetric curves of PLA (a), P75 (b), P50 (c), P25 (d), PCL (f).

The TGA curves of pristine PCL, PLA and their mixtures (as representative of the composite samples too) are showed in Figure 13. It appears that the presence of increasing amount of PLA in the mixtures anticipates either the midpoint degradation or the inflection point of PCL due to the lower degradation temperature of PLA. The introduction of the AMOX does not produce further relevant decrease in the degradation temperature (Table 2). Table 2 contains the main calorimetric data obtained from the heating run of all electrospun samples.

Drug Release Studies

Local release of drugs sustained for many days is preferred to systemic administration due to the advantages of thesedelivery systems, such as: (i) improving the effectiveness of drug and selective targeting; (ii) decreasing the side effects; (iii) reducing the frequency of administration. Therefore following the encapsulation procedures of an antibiotic molecule into a biocompatible polymer, it is of utmost importance to investigate the release profiles, depending on the many parameters that it is possible to modulate for the specific applications. The most important parameters that it is possible to modulate for a local controlled release from elecrospun membranes can be considered: (a) drug concentration; (b) drug location (inside and/or outside the fibers); (c) diameter of the fibers, which in turn determines the membrane porosity and membrane thickness; (d) biodegradation time of the polymeric matrix, that can be quicker than drug diffusion or can simultaneously occur, contributing to the delivery.

Figure 14 [38] shows the release of AMOX at different concentrations from PCL/AMOX membranes, monitored up to 40 days as a function of absolute concentration (*Ct* , mg/L) (Figure 14a) and as percentage of the maximum achievable concentration (Figure 14b). All curves present mainly two stages: a first stage, quick as a "burst," followed by a successive slow second stage. Release kinetics were examined by Korsmeyer-Peppas equation:

$$Q_t/Q_\infty = K_k\, t^n \tag{1}$$

where Q_t/Q_∞ is the drug fraction released at time t, K_k is a constant depending on the structural and geometric characteristic of the system, n is the diffusional coefficient related to the release mechanism.

Higuchi equation was also used:

$$\%Q_t = K_H \tag{2}$$

where $\%Q_t$ is the amount in % of drug released in time t, K_H is the constant depending on the design variables of the system. The calculated kinetic release parameters are show in Table 3.

The initial burst, found in many controlled-release systems for AMOX [21, 40] has been described as caused by a number of mechanisms, including surface desorption, pore diffusion, or the lack of a diffusion front barrier regulating the diffusive process. For customized release processes it must be carefully addressed and controlled, since, depending on application, it may be an optimal mechanism of delivery, as in wound treatment, whereas in others it is undesirable, since the drug can exceed the toxic limits.

Table 3. Initial burst effect and kinetic parameters of AMOX release from PCL electrospun nanofibers using Korsmeyer-Peppas and Higuchi equation

Sample	Initial burst (%)		Korsmeyer-Peppas parameters				Higuchi parameters	
			k_k	n	r^2		k_H	r^2
PCL-A3	41.53		0.374	0.132	0.996		1.952	0.950
PCL-A5	35.65		0.314	0.128	0.983		1.222	0.924
PCL-A7	27.80		0.272	0.126	0.994		1.149	0.933
PCL-A5M3	31.08		0.255	0.122	0.997		1.042	0.929
PCL-A5M6	28.80		0.253	0.124	0.989		1.073	0.933

For the delivery of antibiotic drugs, a initial burst is actually ideal since it is important to eliminate the intruding bacteria before they begin to proliferate. However, for the few organisms that may survive the initial burst, a continued release of antibiotic is necessary to prevent their further population [19, 41, 42].

For investigating the influence of the membrane thickness, samples of PCL-A7 with different thickness 30, 45, 60 μm were prepared. Figure 15 [38] shows the release profiles of AMOX as absolute concentration (*Ct* , mg/L) (Figure 15a) and as percentage of the maximun achievable concentration (Figure 15b). The three curves show the same behavior, which is an initial burst, followed by a slower release. However the initial burst decreases on increasing the membrane thickness, as% respect to the maximum quantity to be delivered, indicating that in this case the burst is mainly a surface phenomenon.

Reporting the percentage of release in the burst, as a function of the membrane thickness a linear behavior that extrapolates to zero for membrane thickness higher than 110 μm was obtained. It can be supposed that for membranes with thickness higher than 110 μm the burst would become irrelevant. This is an important result to control the burst. The second stage release kinetics was examined by Korsmeyer-Peppas equation (Eq. (1)) and Higuchi equations (Eq. (2)): The largest r^2 values were obtained for the Korsmeyer-Peppas equations, with values of n from 0.122 to 0.132. Because of AMOX release present two stages, all formulations followed non-Fickian diffusion mechanism. In the second stage release was attributed mainly to the diffusion or permeation of the drug through PCL matrix.

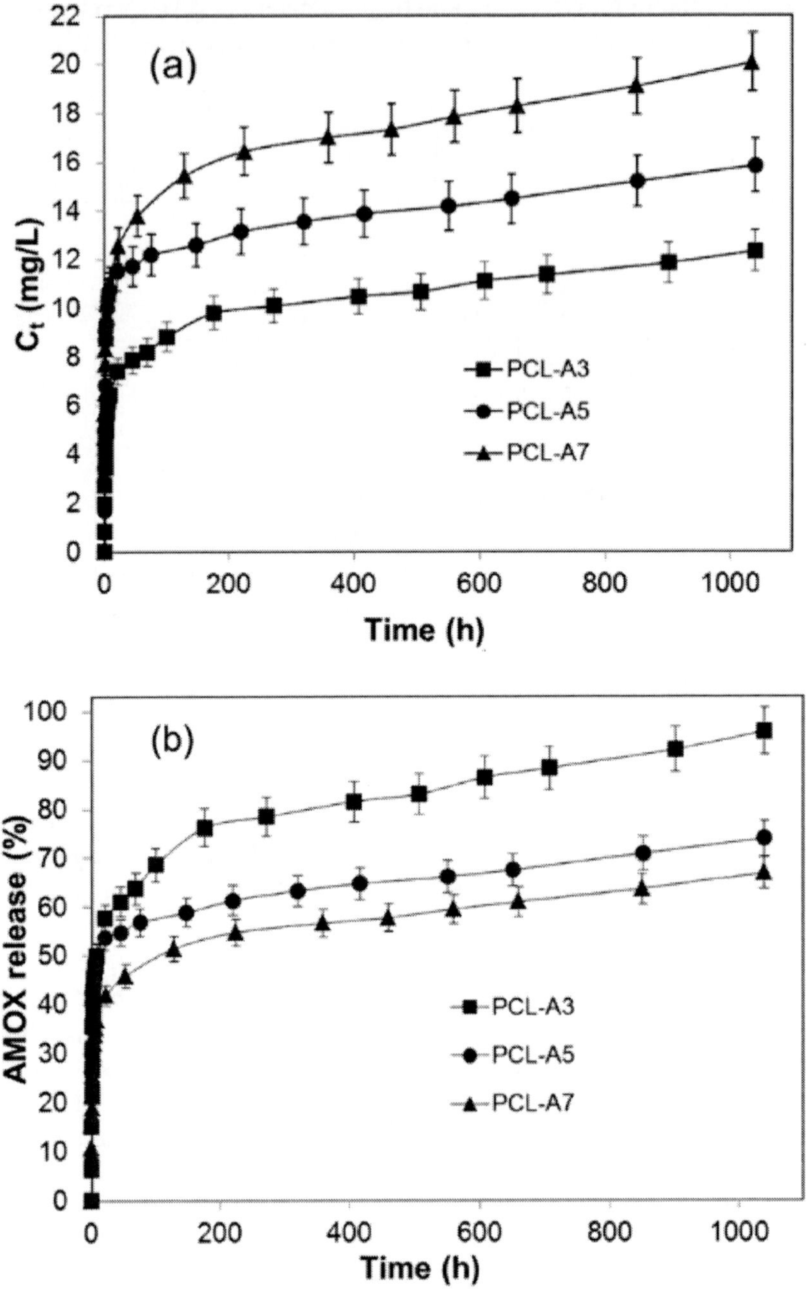

Figure 14. In vitro release profiles of AMOX from PCL-A3, PCL-A5 and PCL-A7, absolute concentration (Ct, mg/L) (a) and as percentage of drug release (b). [38]

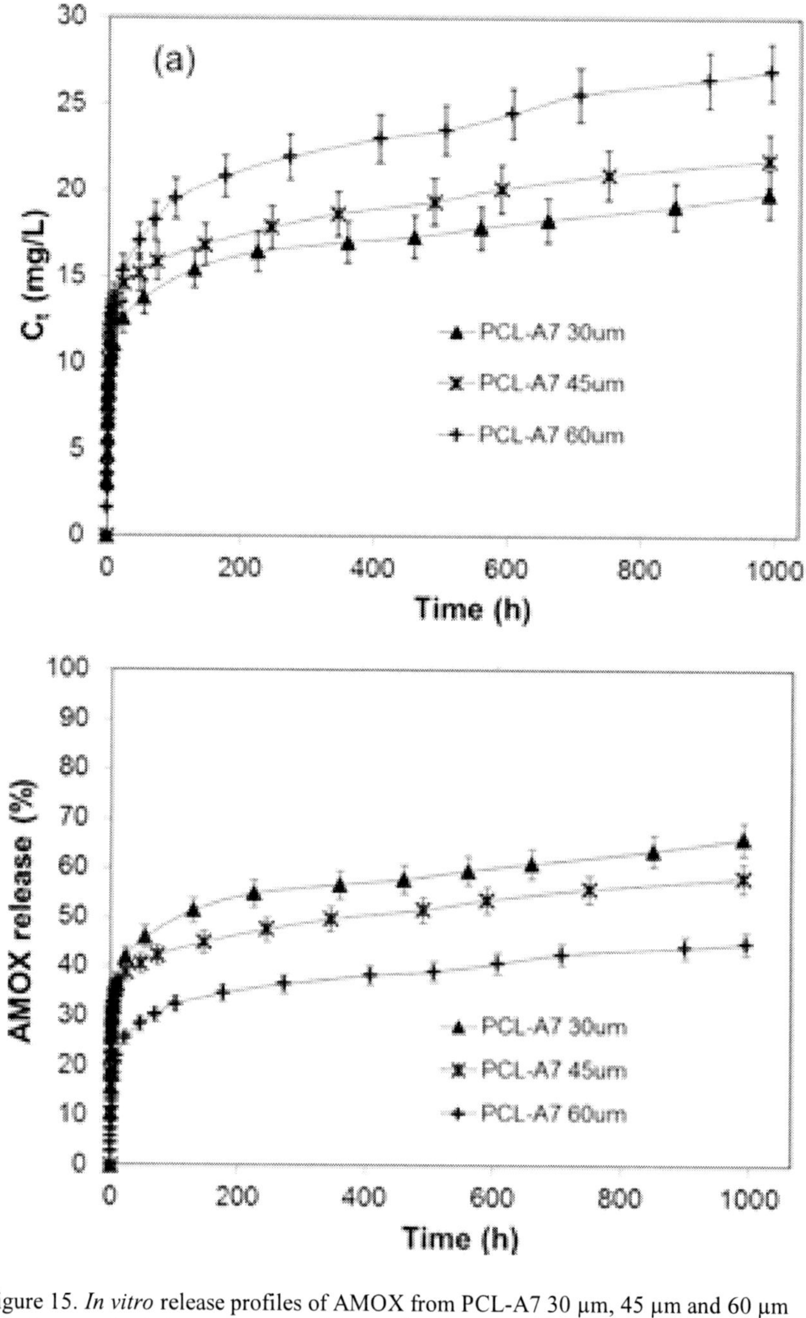

Figure 15. *In vitro* release profiles of AMOX from PCL-A7 30 μm, 45 μm and 60 μm membranes, absolute concentration (Ct , mg/L) (a) and as percentage drug release (b). [38]

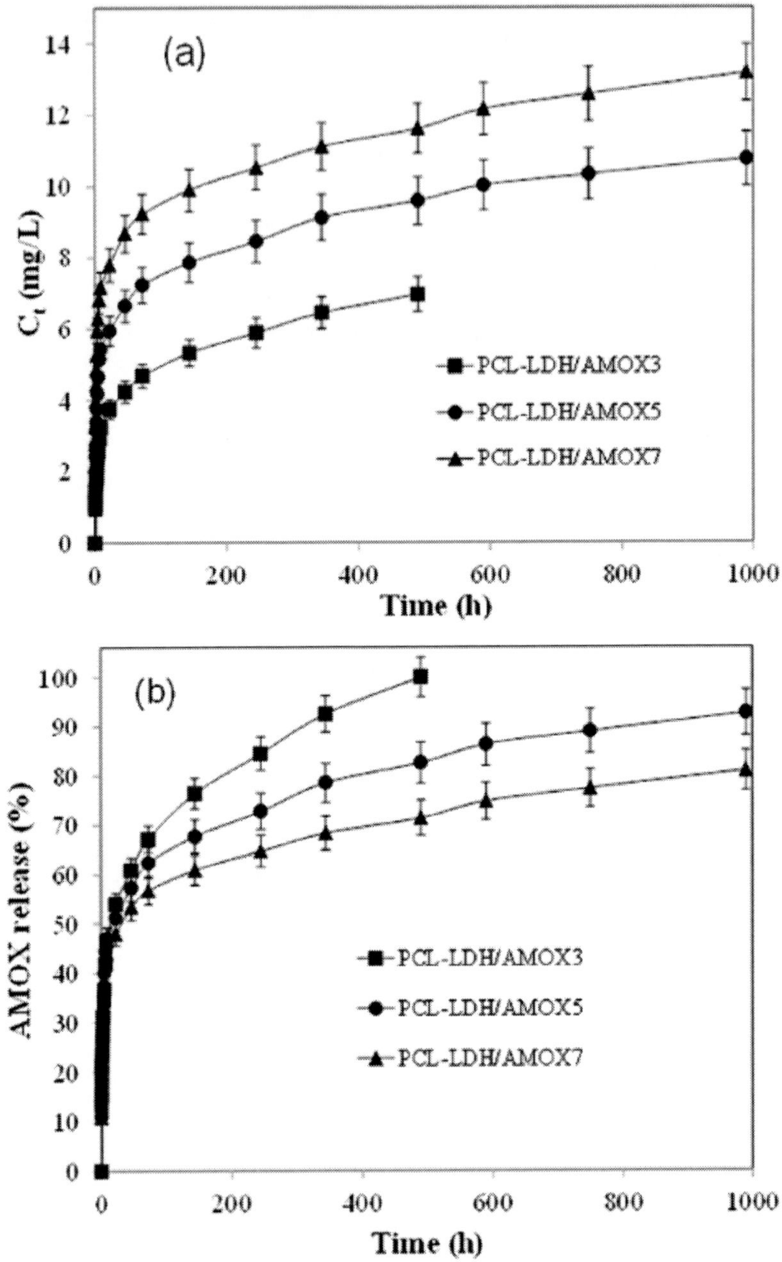

Figure 16. Amount of AMOX released, as absolute concentration (Ct, mg/L) (a) and as % of the maximum achievable concentration (b). Reprinted from Applied Clay Science, 72, Valarezo, E. et. al., 104-109, 2012 [39], with permission from Elsevier.

In Figure 16 [39] the release of AMOX at different concentrations from PCL-LDH/AMOX membranes, monitored up to 40 days, is shown, as absolute concentration (Ct,mg/L) (a) and as % of the maximum achievable concentration (b). The membranes have the same thickness (45 μm) and the same weight and dimensions, and therefore the maximum quantity of amoxicillin present in the nano-hybrid to be released was calculated. In this case an exchange reaction is necessarily followed by a diffusion phenomenon for the AMOX to be released.

As in the case of PCL membranes loaded with pristine AMOX all curves present mainly two stages: a first stage, quick as a "burst", followed by a successive slow second stage. This initial high-rate drug release could be caused by the quick release of LDH/AMOX molecules that should be deposited on the surface area of fibers. After the initial burst an increase of AMOX release, linear with time and extending formany days, depending on LDH/AMOX concentration inside the membrane, was observed. For example the complete release of AMOX from PCL-LDH/AMOX3 is observed after 20 days, whereas it is not yet completed for PCL-LDH/AMOX5 (82%) and PCL-LDH/AMOX7 (71%).

Figure 17 shows the release profiles of AMOX from fibrous PLA/PCL blend mats containing 3, 5 and 7%w/w of drug. Samples showed a sustained release behavior, although an initial rapid drug release was found within the first 8 h.

Also in this case the second stage shows a slow drug release which is attributed mainly to the diffusion or permeation of the drug molecules through polymer matrix towards the release medium.

Release kinetics were examined by equations (1) and (2) and the calculated kinetic release parameters are show in Table 4.

The best r^2 values were obtained for the Higuchi equations. The release constants depend on the AMOX content and polymer concentration. The rate of release increases with increasing of the drug concentration and with the PCL content in the fibers.

Table 4 also shows the amount (%) of AMOX released in the first 500 hours. The releasedpercentages of AMOX increase with both the drug concentration and PCL content in theblend, as expected from the very different amounts released at 500 hours in PLA and PCL(12.94% for PLA-A3 and 83.05% for PCL-A3).

Figure 18 shows the amount of AMOX, released in 500 hours from samples loaded with 3% (a) and 5% of AMOX (b), as a function of phase composition of the blends.

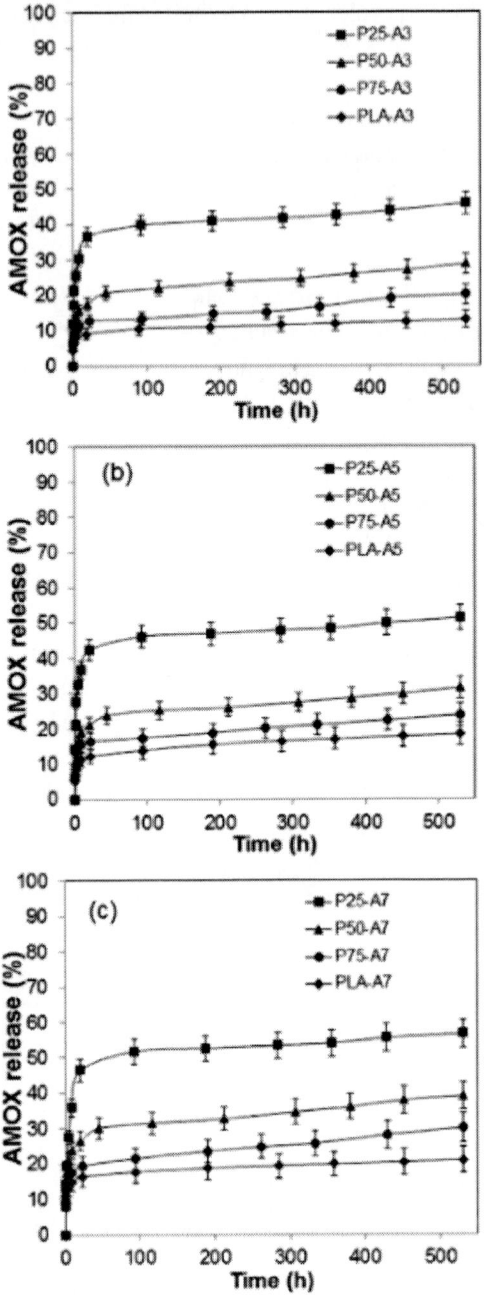

Figure 17. In vitro release profiles from PLA/PCL electrospum membranes loaded with 3% (a), 5% (b) and 7% (c) of AMOX.

Table 4. Kinetic parameters and release amount of AMOX in 500 h for PLA, PCL and PLA/PCL electrospun membranes

Sample	Korsmeyer-Peppas parameters			Higuchi Parameters		Released amount of amoxicillin (%) t=500 h
	k_k	n	r^2	k_H	r^2	
PLA-A3	0.067	0.096	0.982	0.200	0.985	12.94
PLA-A5	0.084	0.116	0.978	0.241	0.998	18.34
PLA-A7	0.095	0.121	0.976	0.343	0.996	20.86
P75-A3	0.077	0.122	0.973	0.387	0.993	20.11
P75-A5	0.099	0.129	0.982	0.418	0.991	23.04
P75-A7	0.113	0.134	0.973	0.466	0.992	29.02
P50-A3	0.112	0.113	0.983	0.435	0.990	25.73
P50-A5	0.122	0.115	0.970	0.438	0.992	27.22
P50-A7	0.156	0.118	0.974	0.545	0.991	33.86
P25-A3	0.253	0.091	0.981	0.513	0.992	45.81
P25-A5	0.302	0.095	0.987	0.532	0.984	50.93
P25-A7	0.324	0.104	0.989	0.557	0.990	55.39
PCL-A3	0.374	0.132	0.996	1.952	0.950	83.05
PCL-A5	0.314	0.128	0.983	1.222	0.924	69.13
PCL-A7	0.272	0.126	0.994	1.149	0.933	59.50

The expected amount of AMOX released from the sample loaded with 3% of AMOX, according to the mixture rule, is:

$$\% \text{ AMOX released} = x\,(12.94) + (1-x)\,(83.05) \quad (3)$$

where x is the content of PLA.

Figure 18 (a) shows that between 100 and 50% of PLA the amount of AMOX vary linearly with PCL content, whereas the dependence at PCL content of 75% is higher. The expected release, according to the mixture rule, is much higher than the experimental. This could be explained with a preferential incorporation of AMOX into PLA, which is a more polar chain respect to PCL.

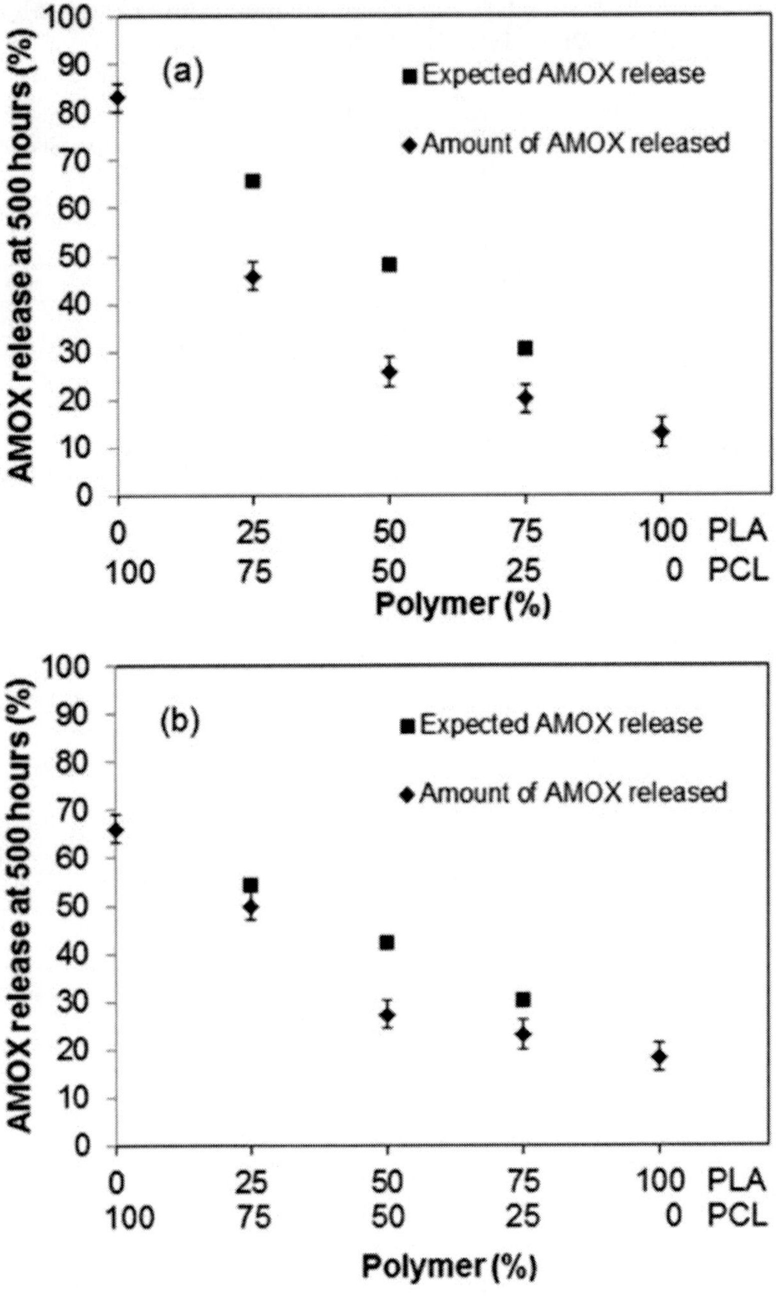

Figure 18. Amount of AMOX released in 500 hours from: PCL-A3 and PLA-A3 (a), PCL-A5 and PLA-A5 (b).

Very similar results are found for the 5% AMOX blends, as shown in Figure 18b. As a matter of fact, the AMOX release is much lower than that expected by the mixture rule for mixtures with 75% and 50% PLA content. Only with 25% of PLA the experimental points are very near to the theoretical points. Evidently, on increasing the AMOX concentration in the mixtures becomes more probable that the drug could be encapsulated also in PCL, in spite of a lower interaction. This is confirmed for the sample with higher AMOX content (7%) (not reported), for which the expected and the calculated values coincide.

Antibacterial Activity *In Vitro*

The inhibitory effect of PCL-A7 against three human pathogenic bacteria by means of disc diffusion, *Staphyococcus aureus*, *Enterococcus faecalis*, and *Escherichia coli* is shown in Figure 19 [38]. The plates (a), (b) and (c), show the inhibition zones, also named inhibition halos around 6 mm discs of PCL-A7. The figure with bigger inhibition zone clearly identifies *S. Aureus* as the most sensible bacteria to AMOX.

Comparing the antibacterial activity of the filled membranes, *S. aureus* results largely the most sensible to AMOX with a maximum of 32.68±0.44 mm, *E. faecalis* shows an intermediate behavior (22.11±0.60 mm) and *E. Coli* is the less inhibited (9.78±0.97 mm) (Table 5).

Less evident is the influence of AMOX concentration, although a slight increase on increasing its concentration can be observed. The explanation can be related to that in the first 24 hours the quantity the AMOX released is similar for all the samples.

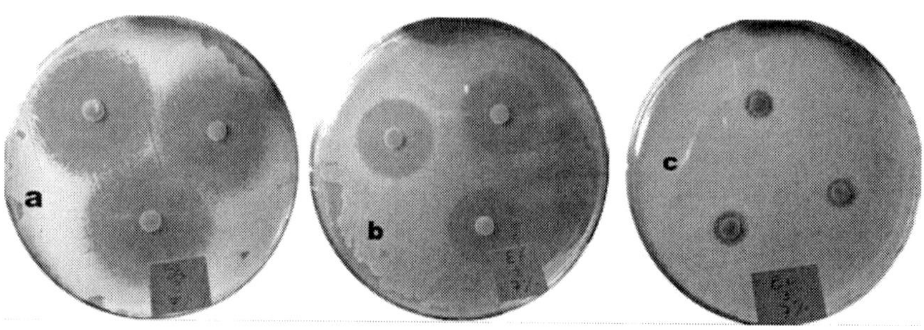

Figure 19. Inhibitory effect of PCL-A7 against three human patogenic bacteria by means of disc diffusion, *Staphyococcus aureus* (a), *Enterococcus faecalis* (b), and *Escherichia coli* (c). [38]

Table 5. Inhibition zone in mm ± SD of AMOX at different concentrations in PCL membranes (the results show the average value of 9 replicates)[38]

Disc diffusion method	*E. coli* (mm ± SD)	*S. aureus* (mm ± SD)	*E. faecalis* (mm ± SD)
PCL-A3	7.67 ± 0.52	30.78 ± 0.44	21.00 ± 0.00
PCL-A5	7.60 ± 0.55	29.78 ± 1.09	20.25 ± 0.46
PCL-A7	9.78 ± 0.97	32.78 ± 0.44	22.11 ± 0.60
PCL	-	-	-
AMOX	20.00 ± 0.00	30.00 ± 0.00	28.00 ± 0.00

Acknowledgments

The corresponding author thanks the Secretaria Nacional de Educación Superior, Ciencia, Tecnología e Innovación of Ecuador for the financial support.

References

[1] Bhardwaj, N., and Kundu, S. C. (2010). Electrospinning: A fascinating fiber fabrication technique. *Biotechnology Advances,* 28, 325-347.

[2] Charernsriwilaiwat, N., Opanasopit, P., Rojanarata, T., Ngawhirunpat, T., and Supaphol, P. (2010). Preparation and characterization of chitosan-hydroxybenzotriazole/polyvinyl alcohol blend nanofibers by the electrospinning technique. *Carbohydrate Polymers,* 81, 675-680.

[3] Chegoonian, P., Feiz, M., Ravandi, S. A. H., and Mallakpour, S. (2012). Preparation of sulfonated poly(ethylene terephthalate) submicron fibrous membranes for removal of basic dyes. *Journal of Applied Polymer Science,* 124, E190-E198.

[4] Chen, H.-C., Tsai, C.-H., and Yang, M.-C. (2011). Mechanical properties and biocompatibility of electrospun polylactide/poly (vinylidene fluoride) mats. *Journal of Polymer Research,* 18, 319-327.

[5] Chong, E. J., Phan, T. T., Lim, I. J., Zhang, Y. Z., Bay, B. H., Ramakrishna, S., and Lim, C. T. (2007). Evaluation of electrospun

PCL/gelatin nanofibrous scaffold for wound healing and layered dermal reconstitution. *Acta Biomaterialia,* 3, 321-330.

[6] Deitzel, J. M., Kleinmeyer, J., Harris, D., and Beck Tan, N. C. (2001). The effect of processing variables on the morphology of electrospun nanofibers and textiles. *Polymer,* 42, 261-272.

[7] Lee, S., and Obendorf, S. K. (2007). Use of Electrospun Nanofiber Web for Protective Textile Materials as Barriers to Liquid Penetration. *Textile Research Journal,* 77, 696-702.

[8] Ribeiro, C., Sencadas, V., Ribelles, J. L. G., and Lanceros-Méndez, S. (2010). Influence of Processing Conditions on Polymorphism and Nanofiber Morphology of Electroactive Poly(vinylidene fluoride) Electrospun Membranes. *Soft Materials,* 8, 274-287.

[9] Greiner, A., and Wendorff, J. H. (2007). Electrospinning: A Fascinating Method for the Preparation of Ultrathin Fibers. *Angewandte Chemie International Edition,* 46, 5670-5703.

[10] Han, J., Branford-White, C. J., and Zhu, L.-M. (2010). Preparation of poly(ε-caprolactone)/poly(trimethylene carbonate) blend nanofibers by electrospinning. *Carbohydrate Polymers,* 79, 214-218.

[11] Huang, X., and Brazel, C. S. (2003). Analysis of burst release of proxyphylline from poly(vinyl alcohol) hydrogels. *Chemical Engineering Communications,* 190, 519-532.

[12] Islam, M. S., and Karim, M. R. (2010). Fabrication and characterization of poly(vinyl alcohol)/alginate blend nanofibers by electrospinning method. *Colloids and Surfaces A: Physicochemical and Engineering Aspects,* 366, 135-140.

[13] Liu, Y., He, J.-H., Yu, J.-y., and Zeng, H.-m. (2008). Controlling numbers and sizes of beads in electrospun nanofibers. *Polymer International,* 57, 632-636.

[14] Ouyang, Y., Huang, C., Zhu, Y., Fan, C., and Ke, Q. (2013). Fabrication of Seamless Electrospun Collagen/PLGA Conduits Whose Walls Comprise Highly Longitudinal Aligned Nanofibers for Nerve Regeneration. *Journal of Biomedical Nanotechnology,* 9, 931-943.

[15] Jaworek, A., Krupa, A., Lackowski, M., Sobczyk, A. T., Czech, T., Ramakrishna, S., Pliszka, D. (2009). Nanocomposite fabric formation by electrospinning and electrospraying technologies. *Journal of Electrostatics,* 67, 435-438.

[16] Sreerekha, P. R., Menon, D., Nair, S. V., and Chennazhi, K. P. Fabrication of Fibrin Based Electrospun Multiscale Composite Scaffold

for Tissue Engineering Applications. *Journal of Biomedical Nanotechnology,* 9, 790-800.

[17] Averous, L., Moro, L., Dole, P., and Fringant, C. (2000). Properties of thermoplastic blends: starch–polycaprolactone. *Polymer,* 41, 4157-4167.

[18] Tan, A., Rajadas, J., and Seifalian, A. M. (2012). Biochemical engineering nerve conduits using peptide amphiphiles. *Journal of Controlled Release,* 163, 342-352.

[19] Kim, K., Luu, Y. K., Chang, C., Fang, D., Hsiao, B. S., Chu, B., and Hadjiargyrou, M. (2004). Incorporation and controlled release of a hydrophilic antibiotic using poly(lactide-co-glycolide)-based electrospun nanofibrous scaffolds. *Journal of Controlled Release,* 98, 47-56.

[20] Lannutti, J., Reneker, D., Ma, T., Tomasko, D., and Farson, D. (2007). Electrospinning for tissue engineering scaffolds. *Materials Science and Engineering: C,* 27, 504-509.

[21] Ahymah Joshy, M. I., Elayaraja, K., Suganthi, R. V., Chandra Veerla, S., and Kalkura, S. N. (2011). In vitro sustained release of amoxicillin from lanthanum hydroxyapatite nano rods. *Current Applied Physics,* 11, 1100-1106.

[22] Songsurang, K., Pakdeebumrung, J., Praphairaksit, N., and Muangsin, N. (2011). Sustained Release of Amoxicillin from Ethyl Cellulose-Coated Amoxicillin/Chitosan–Cyclodextrin-Based Tablets. *AAPS Pharm. Sci. Tech,* 12, 35-45.

[23] Tammaro, L., Costantino, U., Bolognese, A., Sammartino, G., Marenzi, G., Calignano, A., Vittoria, V. (2007). Nanohybrids for controlled antibiotic release in topical applications. *International Journal of Antimicrobial Agents,* 29, 417-423.

[24] Tammaro, L., Costantino, U., Nocchetti, M., and Vittoria, V. (2009). Incorporation of active nano-hybrids into poly(ε-caprolactone) for local controlled release: Antifibrinolytic drug. *Applied Clay Science,* 43, 350-356.

[25] Sammartino, G., Marenzi, G., Tammaro, L., Bolognese, A., Calignano, A., Costantino, U., Vittoria, V. (2005). Anti-inflammatory drug incorporation into polymeric nano-hybrids for local controlled release. *International journal of immunopathology and pharmacology,* 18, 55-62.

[26] Aguzzi, C., Cerezo, P., Viseras, C., and Caramella, C. (2007). Use of clays as drug delivery systems: Possibilities and limitations. *Applied Clay Science,* 36, 22-36.

[27] Cavani, F., Trifirò, F., and Vaccari, A. (1991). Hydrotalcite-type anionic clays: Preparation, properties and applications. *Catalysis Today,* 11, 173-301.

[28] Costantino, U., Marmottini, F., Nocchetti, M., and Vivani, R. (1998). New Synthetic Routes to Hydrotalcite-Like Compounds – Characterisation and Properties of the Obtained Materials. *European Journal of Inorganic Chemistry, 1998*, 1439-1446.

[29] Costantino, U., Ambrogi, V., Nocchetti, M., and Perioli, L. (2008). Hydrotalcite-like compounds: Versatile layered hosts of molecular anions with biological activity. *Microporous and Mesoporous Materials,* 107, 149-160.

[30] Leroux, F., and Taviot-Gueho, C. (2005). Fine tuning between organic and inorganic host structure: new trends in layered double hydroxide hybrid assemblies. *Journal of Materials Chemistry,* 15, 3628-3642.

[31] Rives, V. (2001). Layered Double Hydroxides: Present and Future. New York (US): Nova Science Publishers Inc.

[32] Xu, Z. P., and Braterman, P. S. (2010). Synthesis, structure and morphology of organic layered double hydroxide (LDH) hybrids: Comparison between aliphatic anions and their oxygenated analogs. *Applied Clay Science,* 48, 235-242.

[33] Ardanuy, M., and Velasco, J. I. (2011). Mg–Al Layered double hydroxide nanoparticles: Evaluation of the thermal stability in polypropylene matrix. *Applied Clay Science,* 51, 341-347.

[34] Clinical and Laboratory Standards Institute. (2006). Performance standards for Antimicrobial Disk Susceptibility Tests; Aproved Standard (Ninth ed.). Pennsylvania: Clinical and Laboratory Standards Institute.

[35] Clinical and Laboratory Standards Institute. (2006). Mhetods for Dilution Antimicrobial Susceptibility Tests for Bacteria that Grow Aerobically; Aproved Standard (Seventh ed.). Pennsylvania: Clinical and Laboratory Standards Institute.

[36] Boyanova, L., Gergova, G., Nikolov, R., Derejian, S., Lazarova, E., Katsarov, N., Krastev, Z. (2005). Activity of Bulgarian propolis against 94 *Helicobacter pylori* strains in vitro by agar-well diffusion, agar dilution and disc diffusion methods. *Journal of Medical Microbiology,* 54 481-483.

[37] Kroiss, J., Kaltenpoth, M., Schneider, B., Schwinger, M.-G., Hertweck, C., Maddula, R. K., Svatoš, A. (2010). Symbiotic streptomycetes provide antibiotic combination prophylaxis for wasp offspring. [10.1038/nchembio.331]. *Nature Chemical Biology,* 6, 261-263.

[38] Valarezo, E., Stanzione, M., Tammaro, L., Cartuche, L., Malagón, O., and Vittoria, V. (2013). Preparation, Characterization and Antibacterial Activity of Poly(ε-caprolactone) Electrospun Fibers Loaded with Amoxicillin for Controlled Release in Biomedical Applications. *Journal of Nanoscience and Nanotechnology,* 13, 1717-1726.

[39] Valarezo, E., Tammaro, L., González, S., Malagón, O., and Vittoria, V. (2013). Fabrication and sustained release properties of poly(ε-caprolactone) electrospun fibers loaded with layered double hydroxide nanoparticles intercalated with amoxicillin. *Applied Clay Science,* 72, 104-109.

[40] Said, S. S., Aloufy, A. K., El-Halfawy, O. M., Boraei, N. A., and El-Khordagui, L. K. (2011). Antimicrobial PLGA ultrafine fibers: Interaction with wound bacteria. *European Journal of Pharmaceutics and Biopharmaceutics,* 79, 108-118.

[41] Cui, W., Li, X., Zhu, X., Yu, G., Zhou, S., and Weng, J. (2006). Investigation of Drug Release and Matrix Degradation of Electrospun Poly (dl-lactide) Fibers with Paracetanol Inoculation. *Bio. Macro. molecules,* 7, 1623-1629.

[42] Lagaron, J. M., Ocio, M. J., and Lopez-Rubio, A. (2012). Antimicrobial Polymers. Hoboken, New Jersey: John Wiley and Sons, Inc.

In: Amoxicillin
ISBN: 978-1-62948-489-1
Editors: W. A. Leary and L. M. Kruse

Chapter II

Amoxicillin: Occurrence, Fate and Effects in Aquatic Systems: A Review

João Rosa[1,2], *Sara Leston*[1,2], *Margarida Nunes*[1,2], *Marco F.L. Lemos*[3], *Miguel A. Pardal*[1] *and Fernando Ramos*[2*]

[1]CFE - Centre for Functional Ecology, Department of Life Sciences, University of Coimbra, Coimbra, Portugal

[2]CEF - Center for Pharmaceutical Studies, Health Sciences Campus, Pharmacy Faculty, University of Coimbra, Azinhaga de Santa Comba, Coimbra, Portugal

[3]ESTM and GIRM - Marine Resources Research Group, Polytechnic Institute of Leiria, Peniche, Portugal

Abstract

Antibiotics have been widely used for some decades. Although these substances are developed to perform a biological effect, little attention has been given to the presence of these pharmaceuticals in the environment, namely in aquatic systems. For instance, frequent use of

* Corresponding author: fjramos@ci.uc.pt.

veterinary antibiotics raise concerns related to direct contamination of water and increase in antibiotic resistance of microorganisms. In the aquatic environment, antibiotics can be dissolved in the water and might affect non-target organisms due to bioaccumulation and biomagnification processes. One group of antibiotics largely used to treat infections caused by susceptible bacteria is the penicillins. The present work addresses an up-to-date review on the occurrence, fate and effects of amoxicillin, the most used antibiotic within the β-lactams class, in aquatic systems. It brings up important questions, regarding the uncertainties related to the behavior of amoxicillin in aquatic systems as well as the risks associated with its occurrence.

Introduction

Since the introduction of penicillin in 1941 that medicine has been using antibiotics to treat infectious diseases. In fact, Martinez and co-workers (2009) stated that antibiotics are one of the most successful family of drugs developed so far to improve human health. Besides, with the present increase in food demands, the use of veterinary pharmaceuticals has become essential for the expanding food industry. The potential spread of diseases along with a growing number of animals in farms has made the use of pharmaceuticals a common practice in order to maintain the economic viability of such industries (Sarmah et al., 2006). The main veterinary medicines commonly used in food-animal agriculture comprise not only antibiotics but also endectocides, antifungals, hormones, growth promoters, anesthetics, tranquilizers and anti-inflammatory agents (Boxall et al., 2003b).

Turning the focus on antibiotics, penicillins are a subclass of β-lactams which have been the most widely used antibiotics for more than 80 years, thus constituting the most important group of these pharmaceuticals (Bailón-Pérez et al., 2008). A decade after its discovery by Alexander Fleming, penicillin G became widely available for clinical use and, according to Kummerer and Henninger (2003), penicillins still account for 50% of the total quantity released by hospital effluents. Within the aminopenicillins subgroup, amoxicillin is usually the drug of choice since it is better absorbed following oral administration. This broad spectrum, semi-synthetic antibiotic differs from the "traditional" penicillins due to the presence of an extra amine group. It is effective against a variety of bacteria including *Escherichia coli, Haemophilus influenzae, Pneumococci, Neisseria gonorrhoeae, Streptococci, Staphylococci*, among others (Bebu et al., 2011). These compounds, however, are susceptible to enzymatic modifications and/or degradation and can be inactivated by bacteria capable of producing β-lactamases or penicillinases (Escudero et al., 1996; Prescott, 2007).

Antibiotics in general have been used not only for preventing and treating animal and plant infections, but also as growth promoters in animal intensive farming and to improve feed efficiency (Singer et al., 2003; Cabello, 2006; Sarmah et al., 2006). One of the main concerns about antibiotics is their continuous input in the environment. In the long run, this may lead to high concentrations and therefore become a potential risk to organisms (Mavronikola et al., 2009). This particular issue has been receiving growing attention during the last years due to the increasing concern about pharmaceuticals and its residues. Since many of these were developed to have a biological effect, they present the necessary properties to bioaccumulate and cause effects in aquatic ecosystems (Halling-Sørensen et al., 1998). In the present chapter, a literature review on the occurrence, fate and effects of amoxicillin in aquatic systems has been conducted, since it represents one of the most widely used pharmaceuticals and its presence in the environment is an emerging problem.

Physico-Chemical Characterization

Amoxicillin, also referred to as Amox, Amoxycillin, Amoxicillin anhydrous, Amoxicillin trihydrate or p-Hydroxyampicillin can be found under several trade names, e.g. Amoxil®, Augmentin®, Dispermox® Trimox® or Clavamox®, depending on its use. It presents the formula $C_{16}H_{19}N_3O_5S$ and the molecular weight of 365.41 g mol^{-1}, being formed by a β-lactam ring and a side chain called D-hidroxiphenilglicin (Adriano et al., 2005) (Figure 1). Amoxicillin maintains the same core structure as other penicillins but differs from them by the presence of an extra amino group, which increases its polarity. Another important characteristic of this antibiotic is its amphoteric nature inducing different forms according to the pH. More specifically, when the pH is low the groups ionized become protonated, and when the pH is high the groups ionized are non-protonated, thus resulting in a negative sign (Adriano et al., 2005).

This reaction happens due to the amine, the carboxylic acid and the phenolic hydroxyl ionizable groups, with pK_a values of 7.49, 2.68 and 9.63, respectively (Smyth et al., 1981; Goddard et al., 1996), present in amoxicillin. As to its solubility, at 20°C this antibiotic is highly soluble in water (3430 mg L^{-1}) as well as in organic solvents (7500 mg L^{-1} for methanol and 3400 mg L^{-1} for ethanol).

Mode of Action and Metabolism

Amoxicillin acts by inhibiting the synthesis of the bacterial cell wall, which protects it from the environment (Bebu et al., 2011). Its specific molecular targets are the penicillin binding proteins (transpeptidases) found on the outside of the cytoplasmic membrane, which are involved in the synthesis and remodeling of the cell wall. In Gram-negative bacteria, amoxicillin induces cell lysis through osmosis, weakened by the loss of their peptidoglycan layer; in Gram-positive bacteria amoxicillin prevents the final peptidoglycan cross-linking that gives peptidoglycan its strength (Prescott, 2007).

There are two major metabolites of amoxicillin considered by the FAO: amoxicilloic acid and diketopiperazine. Both compounds lack the antibacterial activity of the parent compound but the amoxicilloic acid can present allergic properties (Reyns et al., 2008; Lamm et al., 2009). As described by Nägele and Moritz (2005), the degradation of amoxicillin in acidic conditions opens the β-lactam ring resulting in the production of amoxicilloic acid. This first product can originate either amoxilloic acid or a new and stable compound, which is diketopiperazine (also called amoxicillin piperazine-2,5-dione or 2,5-diazacyclohexane-1,4-dione, $C_4H_6N_2O_2$). In fact, this chemically stable form of amoxicillin has been found in environmental matrices (Lamm et al., 2009; Pérez-Parada et al., 2011; Gozlan et al., 2013). Furthermore, the amoxicillin molecule can be hydrolyzed, in the presence of a mineral acid and heat, in 2-Amino-2-(p-hydroxyphenyl) acetic acid (Andreozzi et al., 2005) or it can undergo a nucleophilic attack on itself, forming 4-hydroxyphenylglycyl amoxicillin (Hou and Poole, 1971; Nägele and Moritz, 2005). These metabolites can be formed and identified under controlled conditions and have also been found in the aquatic environment. Furthermore, amoxicilloic acid methyl ester metabolite can be formed when a methanol solution is used as eluent in the monitoring of amoxicillin (Grujic et al., 2007; Pérez-Parada et al., 2011). Like other biologically active substances, amoxicillin can enter environmental matrices as the parent compound or its metabolites.

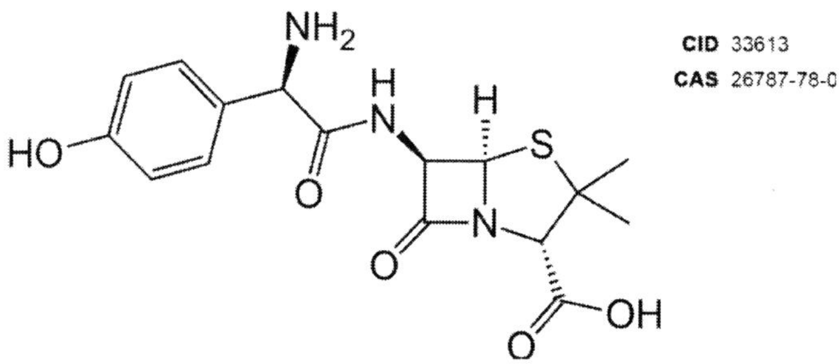

Figure 1. Amoxicillin chemical structure ((2S,5R,6R)-6-[(2R)-2-amino-2-(4-hydroxyphenyl)-acetyl]amino]-3,3-dimethyl-7-oxo-4-thia-1-azabicyclo[3.2.0] heptane-2-carboxylic acid).

Environmental Sources, Fate and Occurrence

β-lactam antibiotics correspond to 50-70% of the total antibiotic use worldwide (Kümmerer, 2009a), and according to the International Medicinal Statistics in 2000, the use of amoxicillin in particular was over 17,000 kg in the UK alone. Its broad-spectrum activity and good absorption rates make amoxicillin one of the most widely used antibiotics.

Medical substances such as amoxicillin can be differentiated into medical substances used by humans, or veterinary medicines, according to types of use, having different exposure routes in the environment. After an internal effect in the human body, amoxicillin will be excreted through urine or faeces, entering the sewage systems and potentially reaching treatment plants (Halling-Sørensen et al., 1998; Kummerer, 2004). Haginaka and Wakai (1987) determined that 67.5% of the dose administrated was excreted in urine - with 49.5% in the unchanged form and 18% as metabolites - but excretion rates up to 80-90% of unmetabolized amoxicillin were also detected (Hirsch et al., 1999; Reviewed by Jjemba, 2006; García-Reiriz et al., 2007). On the other hand, amoxicillin is also used in veterinary medicine where its action can be either for prophylaxis or therapeutic purposes (Halling-Sørensen et al., 1998; Sarmah et al., 2006). Although the majority of the studies report the occurrence of human pharmaceuticals, animal antibiotics have also been found in surface and ground waters (Sarmah et al., 2006), since they may either end up in soil or sediment or in ground waters, essentially when manure is applied to soils (Kummerer, 2004). Amoxicillin can also be found in effluents from drug manufacturing facilities (with effluent loads sometimes reaching several hundreds of milligrams per liter), which until recently were thought to be of minor importance (Kümmerer, 2009a).

Presently, and due to the world growth in the last decades, aquaculture is also a major source of antibiotics in aquatic environments, with amoxicillin being used in the treatment of bacterial infections and as a replacement for antibiotics already suspended by regulatory agencies, such as chloramphenicol (Barnes et al., 1995; FAO, 1999; Serrano, 2005). Amoxicillin used in aquaculture is introduced directly to receiving waters by uneaten feeds as it can leach from the pellets. These pellets are often excessive and will reach the bottom in and around the ponds (Halling-Sørensen et al., 1998). Also, oral absorption of amoxicillin has been reported to be considerably lower for fish than for homeothermic animals (Rocca et al., 2004). The same study also showed very low concentrations of amoxicillin in seabream serum through time, indicating that large amounts are excreted almost directly to water.

Amoxicillin in particular may not be detected in the aquatic environment (Hirsch et al., 1999; Calamari et al., 2003; Palmer et al., 2008), possibly because the residue levels are in very low concentrations, thus requiring more sophisticated analytical tools (Lamm et al., 2009; Mavronikola et al., 2009) or even due to penicillins β-lactam ring high susceptibility to hydrolysis (Hou and Poole, 1971; Deshpande et al., 2004; Lamm et al., 2009; Längin et al., 2009; Mavronikola et al., 2009). For example, when used in aquaculture with a treatment dose of 160 mg kg^{-1}, amoxicillin presented a peak of 531 μg L^{-1} but after 24h would have dissipated and be undetectable (Boxall et al., 2006). In fact, amoxicillin has a heavy environmental load, but it is easily degraded in the environment during several biological and physico-chemical processes (Watkinson et al., 2007), taking only less than 2 days to decrease 90% of its initial concentration, at ambient temperature (Concannon et al., 1986). The persistence of amoxicillin in water matrices is also dependent on pH, being more hydrolyzed at both acidic and alkaline conditions (half life time of 46.1, 19.7, 14.4 and 6.2 d for pH 5, 7, 9 and 3, respectively; Braschi et al., 2013). Identically, Chadha and colleagues (2003) revealed that amoxicillin is more stable at pH 5, with a half-life time of 14.5 d.

To our best knowledge, it has not been clearly stated whether β-lactams were not present in soil, sediments, sludge or slurry, or whether they were simply not analyzed, with few exceptions such as in Zuccato and co-workers (2010), where no amoxicillin was detected in sludge after UV light treatment in an Italian (Varese) sewage treatment plant. Nevertheless, this drug is often found in aquatic environments, mainly through sewage treatment plants which can ultimately discharge this antibiotic into running waters. A review of amoxicillin concentrations found worldwide is presented in table 1. Its low value of octanol-water partition coefficient (Log K_{ow} = 0.87 at pH 7, 20°C; Ramos and colleagues, 2012) indicates that after being administrated and released to the environment, amoxicillin will remain in the aqueous phases, since the higher the Log K_{ow} the higher the probability a residue has to bind to organic matter. To our knowledge, no data about the bioaccumulation potential of amoxicillin was found.

Effects to Aquatic Organisms

Amoxicillin represents potential risks to the aquatic environment, since it has high probability of entering these systems and is widely used (Boxall et al., 2003a; 2003b). For example, the theoretical environmental load of amoxicillin in 2001 in Italy was over 125,000 kg (Calamari et al., 2003). Ecotoxicological tests for single organisms to amoxicillin are presented in table 2. Several other studies are also reviewed in the present chapter, including the effect of antibiotics joint toxicities, using luminescent bacterium assays as an indicator (Ji et al., 2013). Synergistic effects were observed in one of the mixtures with amoxicillin (together with ethanol, acetate, propionate, butyrate, kanamycin, lincomycin and ciprofloxacin), and additive effects were observed in the other (mixture with ethanol, acetate, propionate, butyrate and amoxicillin). By correlating luminescence and the concentration of the pharmaceuticals, the same study determined amoxicillin as the most toxic antibiotic to *Vibrio fischeri* bioluminescence. Similarly, amoxicillin was the most toxic against oral *Actinomyces*, a Gram-positive and filamentous bacteria (LeCorn et al., 2007). Such results were expected, since amoxicillin is a broad spectrum antibiotic with proved efficiency against several types of bacteria (Bebu et al., 2011). Nevertheless, Andreozzi and co-workers (2004) experiments have demonstrated that the unicellular microalgae *Pseudokirchneriella subcapitata* is insensitive to amoxicillin at concentrations ranging from 50 ng L^{-1} to 50 mg L^{-1}. Other experiments performed in the same study did not detect toxicity to *Closterium ehrenbergii*, a large green freshwater algae used to monitor chemical pollution. On the other hand amoxicillin had a marked toxicity for the blue-green algae *Synechococcus leopolensis* (NOEC=0.78 μg L^{-1}; LOEC=1.56 μg L^{-1}; $EC_{50,96h}$=2.22 μg L^{-1}). In general, the second most sensitive organisms are probably cyanobacteria, due to their structure, which is very similar to bacteria (Lützhøft et al., 1999). Moreover, González-Pleiter and co-workers (2013) obtained the same results, indicating that amoxicillin did not present any toxicity to the green algae used, but for the cyanobacteria *Anabaena* sp. the concentrations of 56.3, 15.1 and 6.16 mg L^{-1} for EC_{50}, EC_{20} and EC_{10}, respectively, inhibited the constitutive luminescence of this organism. These authors concluded that certain antibiotic mixtures may pose an ecological risk for aquatic ecosystems, with concentrations already measured in the environment. Also, in the mg L^{-1} range, amoxicillin evidently affected the photosynthetic activity of *Synechocystis* sp. (namely the photosystem II), with the toxic effect increasing with increasing amoxicillin concentrations (Pan et al., 2008). These results were in accordance with the work from Opriş and others (2013). Amoxicillin (in the range of mg L^{-1}) reduced not only the chlorophyll content of the common wheat *Triticum aestivum* but also the capacity of light reactions of photosynthesis, which can ultimately impair photosynthesis under lower light conditions (Opriş et al., 2013). Experiments carried out with the sedentary cnidarian *Hydra vulgaris*, a freshwater invertebrate already used for studying freshwater pollutants, showed no toxicity of amoxicillin in the concentrations tested (10, 100 µg L^{-1}, 1.0, 10 mg L^{-1}) for feeding and polyp regeneration. However, concentrations higher than 100 µg L^{-1} induced effects in the polyp structure, according to a grade scoring system of its morphological status (Pascoe et al., 2003). Studies with higher ecological relevance were also performed using amoxicillin. For instance, Çelebi and Sponza (2012) assessed the acute toxicity of three trophic levels in a laboratory-scale anaerobic multi-chamber bed reactor system, simulating a sewage treatment plant. These authors determined the toxicity before and after the treatment of the sludge, with an initial concentration of 150 mg L^{-1} of amoxicillin. They obtained a maximum of 94% removal of amoxicillin and the EC_{50} values increased from 143 to 248.5, 97 to 281.5, and 210 to 332.5 mg L^{-1} for *Vibrio fischeri*, *Daphnia magna*, and the fish *Lepistes* sp., respectively. These results are not in absolute accordance to the findings of Park and Choi (2008), who determined the toxicity of amoxicillin to a marine bacteria, two cladocerans and a fish species. Only the bacteria, *V. fischeri*, was affected when exposed to amoxicillin ($EC_{50,15min}$=3600 mg L^{-1}), while *D. magna*, *Moina macrocopa* and *Oryzias latipes* were not affected by the tested concentrations. With the intent to study the effect of pharmaceuticals in fish, Laville and co-workers (2004) tested several classes of pharmaceuticals on two fish hepatocyte models: primary cultures of rainbow trout hepatocytes and PLHC-1 fish cell line. Amoxicillin did not present any cytotoxicity at concentrations up to 500 µM.

Table 1. Dissolved amoxicillin and metabolites concentrations (ng L^{-1}) present in natural water samples

Country	Location	Aquatic system	Collecting period	Compound	Detection frequency (%)	Mean concentration (ng L^{-1})	Maximum concentration (ng L^{-1})	Reference
Australia	Queensland	Hospital wastewater	Feb 2005-Jul2006	Amoxicillin	100	90	900	Watkinson et al., 2009
	Queensland	STP influent	Feb 2005-Jul2006	Amoxicillin	89	1400	6940	Watkinson et al., 2009
	Queensland	STP effluent	Feb 2005-Jul2006	Amoxicillin	4	-	50	Watkinson et al., 2009
	Queensland	Surface waters	Feb 2005-Jul2006	Amoxicillin	30	-	200	Watkinson et al., 2009
	Brisbane	STP influent	2006	Amoxicillin		190	280	Watkinson et al., 2007
China	Hong Kong (4 locations)	STP effluent	Jun-Aug 2008	Amoxicillin	57.2	696.4	1670	Minh et al., 2009
	Victoria harbor, Hong Kong	Sea water	Jun-Aug 2008	Amoxicillin	90.0	15.9	128	Minh et al., 2009
	Hong Kong	STP influent	Jun-Aug 2008	Amoxicillin	71.4	511.2	1550	Leung et al., 2012
	Hong Kong	STP effluent	Jun-Aug 2008	Amoxicillin	71.4	700	1868	Leung et al., 2012
France	Paris	Seine River	Dec 2009	Amoxicillin		68	-	Tuc Dinh et al., 2011
Italy	Palermo, Latina, Varese Olona	STP effluent	Jan-Fev 2004	Amoxicillin	37.5	53.3	120	Castiglioni et al., 2005
	Cagliari, Palermo, Roma, Napoli, Torino, Varese Olona, Varese Lago	STP effluent	2004	Amoxicillin	87.5	22.7	120.4	Andreozzi et al., 2004
	Varese	STP influent	2007-2008	Amoxicillin	-	18	-	Zuccato et al., 2010
	Northern Italy (4 locations)	Po River	2007-2008	Amoxicillin	-	< 2.08	-	Zuccato et al., 2010

Table 1. (Continued)

Country	Location	Aquatic system	Collecting period	Compound	Detection frequency (%)	Mean concentration (ng L^{-1})	Maximum concentration (ng L^{-1})	Reference
	Central Italy (4 locations)	Arno River	2007-2008	Amoxicillin	-	5.7	9.9	Zuccato et al., 2010
Israel	Glil Yam	STP effluent	2011	Amoxicillin penilloic acid	-	150	-	Gozlan et al., 2013
	Glil Yam	STP effluent	2011	Diketopiperazine	-	500	-	Gozlan et al., 2013
	Glil Yam	Groundwater	2011	Diketopiperazine	-	30	-	Gozlan et al., 2013
	Sharon Region (18 STP)	STP influent	Fev-Mar 2008	Diketopiperazine	100.0	< LOQ	-	Lamm et al., 2009
	Sharon Region (18 STP)	STP effluent	Fev-Mar 2008	Diketopiperazine	100.0	< LOQ	-	Lamm et al., 2009
Poland	Poznan	Warta River	Jan 2007	Amoxicillin	-	< LOQ	-	Kasprzyk-Hordern et al., 2007
UK	Wales	Taff River	Dec 2006	Amoxicillin	75.0	107.8	245	Kasprzyk-Hordern et al., 2007
	Wales	Taff River	Nov 2006-Aug 2007	Amoxicillin	73.8	125.5	622	Kasprzyk-Hordern et al., 2008

Table 2. Ecotoxicity values for aquatic organisms exposed to amoxicillin - parent compound

Group	Species	Endpoint and exposure time		Concentration (µg L^{-1})	Reference
Freshwater					
(Cyanobacteria)	*Microcystis aeruginosa*	Growth	$EC_{50,7d}$	3.7	Lützhøft et al., 1999
	M. aeruginosa	Growth	$EC_{50,7d}$	8.03	Liu et al., 2012
	Synechococcus leopoliensis	Growth	$EC_{50,96h}$	2.22	Andreozzi et al., 2004
	Anabaena sp.[b]	Bioluminescence	$EC_{50,72h}$	56,300	González-Pleiter et al., 2013
	Anabaena sp.[b]	Bioluminescence	$EC_{20,72h}$	15,100	González-Pleiter et al., 2013
	Anabaena sp.[b]	Bioluminescence	$EC_{10,72h}$	61,600	González-Pleiter et al., 2013
(Chlorophyte)	*Selenastrum capricornutum*[c]	Growth	$NOEC_{7d}$	250,000	Lützhøft et al., 1999
	Pseudokirkneriella subcapitata	Growth	$EC_{50,72h}$	> $1.5x10^6$	González-Pleiter et al., 2013
	P. subcapitata	Growth	$EC_{20,72h}$	> $1.5x10^6$	González-Pleiter et al., 2013
	P. subcapitata	Growth	$EC_{10,72h}$	> $1.5x10^6$	González-Pleiter et al., 2013
Aquatic plant	*Lemna gibba*	Wet weight, Frond number, Carotenoids, Chlorophyll *a* and *b*	$EC_{50,7d}$	> 1,000	Brain et al., 2004
	L. gibba	Wet weight, Frond number, Carotenoids, Chlorophyll *a* and *b*	$EC_{25,7d}$	> 1,000	Brain et al., 2004

Table 2. (Continued)

Group	Species	Endpoint and exposure time		Concentration ($\mu g\ L^{-1}$)	Reference
	L. gibba	Wet weight, Frond number, Carotenoids, Chlorophyll *a* and *b*	$EC_{10,7d}$	> 1,000	Brain et al., 2004
	Daphnia magna	Growth and reproduction	$EC_{50,24h}$	> $1.0x10^6$	Park and Choi, 2008
	D. magna	Growth and reproduction	$EC_{50,48h}$	> $1.0x10^6$	Park and Choi, 2008
	Moina macrocopa	Growth and reproduction	$EC_{50,24h}$	> $1.0x10^6$	Park and Choi, 2008
	M. macrocopa	Growth and reproduction	$EC_{50,48h}$	> $1.0x10^6$	Park and Choi, 2008
Marine					
	Vibrio fischeri	Bioluminescence	$IC_{50,5min}$	$1.32x10^6$	Park and Choi, 2008
	V. fischeri	Bioluminescence	$IC_{50,15min}$	$3.6x10^6$	Park and Choi, 2008
Algae	*Rhodomonas salina*	Growth	$EC_{50,3d}$	$3.1x10^6$ [a]	Lützhøft et al., 1999
Fish	*Oryzias latipes*	Mortality	$LC_{50,24h}$	> $1.0x10^6$	Park and Choi, 2008
	O. latipes	Mortality	$LC_{50,48h}$	> $1.0x10^6$	Park and Choi, 2008

[a] out of measured range.

[b] Anabaena sp. PCC 7120 strain CPB4337.

[c] former name to *Pseudokirchneriella subcapitata.*

One major aspect of concern nowadays is the resistance acquired to different antimicrobials. The problem associated may not be the concentrations found in environmental samples, but the continuous input of amoxicillin. It is known that resistant bacteria are favored by the presence of antibiotics at sub-therapeutic concentrations, for a long period of time (Kümmerer, 2009b). These authors state that the input of resistant bacteria is even more alarming than the input of antibiotics itself, and it can be transmitted to humans by direct contact from animals, through the food chain or via contaminated water/soil. Amoxicillin can be administrated individually, but can also be used as a mass treatment, via feed or drinking water (or directly in water, in the case of aquaculture production). It can also be administrated together with other pharmaceuticals, like the amoxicillin-clavulanic acid, which is a combination of this antibiotic with a β-lactamase inhibitor. The risk of developing resistance increases when antibiotics are intended for group medication (Belmar-Liberato et al., 2011). An extensive literature review on resistance to amoxicillin in animals in Europe is presented by Belmar-Liberato and co-workers (2011), with several cases of not only amoxicillin but also amoxicillin-clavulanic resistance detected in several countries.

Regulation and Legislation

In the last decades, there has been a change in how the world looks at human and animal welfare. Now, more than ever, there is a holistic approach to guarantee the safe use of antibiotics in human medicine as well as in the animal production sector. In this sense, several legislations and regulations have been approved, setting principles to ensure the safe administration of such compounds. In the EU, Regulation (EC) 470/2009 laid down the procedures to establish the residue limits for pharmacologically active substances while taking into account risk assessment and risk management (EC Regulation 470/2009). This document was based on the previous Regulation (EC) 2377/90 which aimed to prevent the hazards associated with the consumption of unsafe residues in edible tissues by establishing their maximum residue levels (MRL) (EC Regulation 2377/90). In 2010, this was replaced by the Commission Regulation (EC) 37/2010, where the compounds are listed alphabetically and sorted into two tables for allowed and prohibited substances, following the guidelines given by Regulation (EC) 470/2009 and their respective MRL (EC Regulation 37/2010).

Regarding the use of amoxicillin in veterinary medicine, it is approved as amoxicillin trihydrate and can be administered in all food-producing species including cattle, pigs, sheep and poultry with specific dosage according to the body weight of the animals. The only exception is applied to egg-producing species to which amoxicillin cannot be given. As for the administration routes, it can be applied in oral suspensions, drench, mixed in milk, in powder form or as an injection suspension either intramuscularly or subcutaneously (Ramos et al., 2012). As such, in order to safeguard the consumers' health, amoxicillin MRLs are established in the Commission Regulation (EC) 37/2010 under the permitted substances included in the Table 1 of that regulation. Accordingly, the MRLs for muscle, fat, liver and kidney are set at 50 µg/kg whereas in milk it is set at 4 µg/kg (EC Regulation 37/2010). These values are based on several parameters that include: i) an acceptable daily intake (ADI) of 0-0.7 µg/kg bw; ii) the lack of microbiological activity of the two major metabolites, amoxicilloic acid and amoxicillin diketopiperazine, which make amoxicillin a suitable marker residue; iii) the highest residues are found in the kidney which acts as a suitable target tissue; iv) existing validated routine analytical methods for monitoring purposes and v) the MRLs are based on twice the LOQ of 25 µg/kg in edible tissues and 2 µg/kg for milk (Ramos et al., 2012).

Conclusion

It was only in the recent years that antibiotics were taken into account in several complex investigations. Despite being used in large quantities for several decades, the existence of these pharmaceuticals in the environment has received little attention until recently, but nowadays the antibiotic contamination scenario concerns not only the environment but also human health. Amoxicillin is a largely used antibiotic to treat bacterial infections caused by several microorganisms, increasing the probability of this antibiotic to reach aquatic systems (Boxall et al., 2003a; 2003b). Nevertheless, as β-lactams may be easily inactivated by the cleavage of the β-lactam ring (Hou and Poole, 1971; Deshpande et al., 2004; Lamm et al., 2009; Längin et al., 2009; Mavronikola et al., 2009), amoxicillin is mainly found on sewage treatment plants or hospital wastewaters, with the exception of few studies where amoxicillin was detected in running waters (e.g. Seine River, Tuc Dinh et al., 2011; Taff River, Kasprzyk-Hordern et al., 2007, 2008; sea water at Hong Kong, Minh et al., 2009). Despite the reports that β-lactam antibiotics are likely to dominate the whole antibiotic concentration in some sewage influents, they tend to be considerably reduced in concentrations during several biological and physic-chemical processes (Watkinson et al., 2007), therefore its concentrations in environmental samples are often minute. Nevertheless, it is known that amoxicillin may be present in aquatic systems and even present toxicity at environmental relevant concentrations. However, many of the studies on pharmaceutical effects found during the present literature review did not include amoxicillin ecotoxicological tests. Such can be either due to the methodologies adopted, or because it is not found in the analyses performed for pharmaceuticals in environmental matrices. Also, all toxicity tests were performed for amoxicillin parent compound, yet some metabolites have been detected in the environment (e.g. Lamm et al., 2009; Gozlan et al., 2013). Furthermore, scientific research on the fate and behavior of antibiotics in soils and sediments is scarce, and to our knowledge inexistent concerning amoxicillin. Since sediments can be identified as major sinks for antibiotics used in aquatic environments (Leston et al, 2011), problems in terrestrial ecosystems such as effects on nitrifying bacteria, growth inhibition of crop plants, and edaphic fauna can occur (Kümmerer, 2009a). Although the effect on bacteria is expected, the interruption of the food web may affect the diversity of a system. There is an increasing concern in public health, related to the effects of the subinhibitory concentrations of antibiotics. The resistance acquired, as well as the transmission of resistant strains may lead to a serious therapeutic problem in human or veterinary medicine (Leston et al., 2011).

Acknowledgments

The authors are grateful for the financial support of the FCT – Fundação para a Ciência e Tecnologia of the Portuguese Government through a fund for RISKFISH project (PTDC/AGR-ALI/122119/2010).

References

Adriano, W. S., Veredas, V., Santana, C. C. & Gonçalves, L. R. B. (2005). Adsorption of amoxicillin on chitosan beads: Kinetics, equilibrium and validation of finite bath models. *Biochemical Engineering Journal*, *27*, 132–137.

Andreozzi, R., Canterino, M., Marotta, R. & Paxeus, N. (2005). Antibiotic removal from wastewaters: The ozonation of amoxicillin. *Journal of Hazardous Materials*, *122*, 243–250.

Andreozzi, R., Caprio, V., Ciniglia, C., de Champdoré, M., Giudice, Lo, R., Marotta, R. & Zuccato, E. (2004). Antibiotics in the environment: occurrence in Italian STPs, fate, and preliminary assessment on algal toxicity of amoxicillin. *Environmental Science & Technology*, *38*, 6832–6838.

Bailón-Pérez, M. I., Garcia-Campaña, A. M., Cruces-Blanco, C. & del Olmo Iruela, M. (2008). Trace determination of β-lactam antibiotics in environmental aqueous samples using off-line and on-line preconcentration in capillary electrophoresis. *Journal of Chromatography A 1185*, 273–280.

Barnes, A. C., Hastings, T. S. & Amyes, S. (1995). Aquaculture antibacterials are antagonized by seawater cations. *Journal of Fish Diseases 18*, 463–465.

Bebu, A., Szabó, L., Leopold, N., Berindean, C. & David, L. (2011). IR, Raman, SERS and DFT study of amoxicillin. *Journal of Molecular Structure*, *993*, 52–56.

Belmar-Liberato, R., Gonzalez-Canga, A., Tamame-Martin, P. & Escribano-Salazar, M. (2011). Amoxicillin and amoxicillin-clavulanic acid resistance in veterinary medicine–the situation in Europe: a review. *Veterinarni Medicina*, *56*, 473–485.

Boxall, A., Fogg, L., Baird, D., Telfer, T., Lewis, C., Gravell, A. & Boucard, T. (2006). Targeted monitoring study for veterinary medicines. Environment Agency R & D Technical Report, Bristol, UK, Environment Agency.

Boxall, A., Fogg, L. A., Kay, P., Blackwel, P. A., Pemberton, E. J. & Croxford, A. (2003)a. Prioritisation of veterinary medicines in the UK environment. *Toxicology Letters*, *142*, 207–218.

Boxall, A. B. A., Kolpin, D. W., Halling-Sørensen, B. & Tolls, J. (2003)b. Are veterinary medicines causing environmental risks? *Environmental Science & Technology*, *37*, 286A–294A.

Brain, R. A., Johnson, D. J., Richards, S. M., Sanderson, H., Sibley, P. K. & Solomon, K. R. (2004). Effects of 25 pharmaceutical compounds to *Lemna gibba* using a seven-day static-renewal test. *Environmental Toxicology and Chemistry*, *23*, 371–382.

Braschi, I., Blasioli, S., Fellet, C., Lorenzini, R., Garelli, A., Pori, M. & Giacomini, D. (2013). Persistence and degradation of new β-lactam antibiotics in the soil and water environment. *Chemosphere*, *93*, 152–159.

Cabello, F. C. (2006). Heavy use of prophylactic antibiotics in aquaculture: a growing problem for human and animal health and for the environment. *Environmental Microbiology*, *8*, 1137–1144.

Calamari, D., Zuccato, E., Castiglioni, S., Bagnati, R. & Fanelli, R. (2003). Strategic Survey of Therapeutic Drugs in the Rivers Po and Lambro in Northern Italy. *Environmental Science & Technology*, *37*, 1241–1248.

Castiglioni, S., Bagnati, R., Calamari, D., Fanelli, R. & Zuccato, E. (2005). A multiresidue analytical method using solid-phase extraction and high-pressure liquid chromatography tandem mass spectrometry to measure pharmaceuticals of different therapeutic classes in urban wastewaters. *Journal of Chromatography As*, *1092*, 206–215.

Chadha, R., Kashid, N. & Jain, D. V. S. (2003). Kinetic studies of the degradation of an aminopenicillin antibiotic (amoxicillin trihydrate) in aqueous solution using heat conduction microcalorimetry. *Archiv für Hydrobiologie*, *55*, 1495–1503.

Concannon, J., Lovitt, H., Ramage, M., Tai, L. H., Mc Donald, C. & Sunderland, V. B. (1986). Stability of aqueous solutions of amoxicillin sodium in the frozen and liquid states. *American Journal of Health-System Pharmacy*, *43*, 3027–3030.

Çelebi, H., Sponza, D. T. (2012). Comparison of the sensitivities of fish, Microtox and *Daphnia magna* bioassays to amoxycillin in anaerobic/ aerobic sequential reactor systems. *Water Science & Technology*, *66*, 1117.

Deshpande, A. D., Baheti, K. G. & Chatterjee, N. R., (2004). Degradation of β-lactam antibiotics. *Current Science*, *87*, 1684–1695.

Escudero, E., Carceles, C. M. & Vicente, S. (1996). Pharmacokinetics of amoxicillin/clavulanic acid combination and of both drugs alone after intravenous administration to goats. *British Veterinary Journal*, *152*, 551–559.

FAO. (1999). Food safety issues associated with products from aquaculture. Report of a Joint FAO/NACA/WHO Study Group. *World Health Organanization Technical Report Series*, *883*, 1–55.

García-Reiriz, A., Damiani, P. C. & Olivieri, A. C. (2007). Different strategies for the direct determination of amoxicillin in human urine by second-order multivariate analysis of kinetic–spectrophotometric data. *Talanta*, *71*, 806–815.

Goddard, A. F., Jessa, M. J., Barrett, D. A., Shaw, P. N., Idström, J. P., Cederberg, C. & Spiller, R. C. (1996). Effect of omeprazole on the distribution of metronidazole, amoxicillin, and clarithromycin in human gastric juice. *Gastroenterology*, *111*, 358–367.

González-Pleiter, M., Gonzalo, S., Rodea-Palomares, I., Leganés, F., Rosal, R., Boltes, K., Marco, E. & Fernández-Piñas, F. (2013). Toxicity of five antibiotics and their mixtures towards photosynthetic aquatic organisms: Implications for environmental risk assessment. *Water Research*, *47*, 2050–2064.

Gozlan, I., Rotstein, A. & Avisar, D. (2013). Amoxicillin-degradation products formed under controlled environmental conditions: Identification and determination in the aquatic environment. *Chemosphere*, *91*, 985–992.

Grujic, S., Vasiljevic, T., Lausevic, M. & Ast, T. (2007). Study on the formation of an amoxicillin adduct with methanol using electrospray ion trap tandem mass spectrometry. *Rapid Communications in Mass Spectrometry*, *22*, 67–74.

Haginaka, J. & Wakai, J. (1987). Liquid chromatographic determination of amoxicillin and its metabolites in human urine by postcolumn degradation with sodium hypochlorite. *Journal of chromatography*, *413*, 219–226.

Halling-Sørensen, B., Nors Nielsen, S., Lanzky, P. F., Ingerslev, F., Holten Lützhøft, H. C. & Jørgensen, S. E., (1998). Occurrence, fate and effects of pharmaceutical substances in the environment-a review. *Chemosphere*, *36*, 357–393.

Hirsch, R., Ternes, T., Haberer, K. & Kratz, K. L. (1999). Occurrence of antibiotics in the aquatic environment. *Science of The Total Environment*, *225*, 109–118.

Hou, J. P. & Poole, J. W. (1971). β-lactam antibiotics: Their physicochemical properties and biological activities in relation to structure. *Journal of Pharmaceutical Sciences*, *60*, 503–532.

Ji, J.-Y., Xing, Y.-J., Ma, Z.-T., Zhang, M. & Zheng, P. (2013). Acute toxicity of pharmaceutical wastewaters containing antibiotics to anaerobic digestion treatment. *Chemosphere*, *91*, 1094–1098.

Jjemba, P. K. (2006). Excretion and ecotoxicity of pharmaceutical and personal care products in the environment. *Ecotoxicology and Environmental Safety*, *63*, 113–130.

Kasprzyk-Hordern, B., Dinsdale, R. M. & Guwy, A. J. (2007). Multi-residue method for the determination of basic/neutral pharmaceuticals and illicit drugs in surface water by solid-phase extraction and ultra performance liquid chromatography–positive electrospray ionisation tandem mass spectrometry. *Journal of Chromatography A*, *1161*, 132–145.

Kasprzyk-Hordern, B., Dinsdale, R. M. & Guwy, A. J. (2008). The occurrence of pharmaceuticals, personal care products, endocrine disruptors and illicit drugs in surface water in South Wales, UK. *Water Research*, *42*, 3498–3518.

Kummerer, K. (2004). Resistance in the environment. *Journal of Antimicrobial Chemotherapy*, *54*, 311–320.

Kummerer, K. & Henninger, A. (2003). Promoting resistance by the emission of antibiotics from hospitals and households into efluent. *Clinical Microbiology and Infection*, *9*, 1203–1214.

Kümmerer, K. (2009)a. Antibiotics in the aquatic environment – A review – Part I. *Chemosphere*, *75*, 417–434.

Kümmerer, K. (2009)b. Antibiotics in the aquatic environment – A review – Part II. *Chemosphere*, *75*, 435–441.

Lamm, A., Gozlan, I., Rotstein, A. & Avisar, D. (2009). Detection of amoxicillin-diketopiperazine-2′, 5′ in wastewater samples. *Journal of Environmental Science and Health, Part A*, *44*, 1512–1517.

Laville, N., Aït-Aïssa, S., Gomez, E., Casellas, C. & Porcher, J. M. (2004). Effects of human pharmaceuticals on cytotoxicity, EROD activity and ROS production in fish hepatocytes. *Toxicology*, *196*, 41–55.

Längin, A., Alexy, R., König, A. & Kümmerer, K. (2009). Deactivation and transformation products in biodegradability testing of ß-lactams amoxicillin and piperacillin. *Chemosphere*, *75*, 347–354.

LeCorn, D. W., Vertucci, F. J., Rojas, M. F., Progulske-Fox, A. & Bélanger, M. (2007). In Vitro Activity of Amoxicillin, Clindamycin, Doxycycline, Metronidazole, and Moxifloxacin Against Oral Actinomyces. *Journal of Endodontics*, *33*, 557–560.

Leston S., Nunes M., Lemos M. F. L., Silva G., Pardal M. A. & Ramos F. (2011). The veterinary drugs use and environmental safety. In: Animal Feed: Types, Nutrition and Safety. Borgearo S.R. (eds) Nova Science Publishers, Inc. New York, 61-83

Leung, H. W., Minh, T. B., Murphy, M. B., Lam, J. C. W., So, M. K., Martin, M., Lam, P. K. S. & Richardson, B. J. (2012). Distribution, fate and risk assessment of antibiotics in sewage treatment plants in Hong Kong, South China. *Environment International*, *42*, 1–9.

Liu, Y., Gao, B., Yue, Q., Guan, Y., Wang, Y. & Huang, L. (2012). Influences of two antibiotic contaminants on the production, release and toxicity of microcystins. *Ecotoxicology and Environmental Safety*, *77*, 79–87.

Lützhøft, H. H., Halling-Sørensen, B. & Jørgensen, S. E. (1999). Algal toxicity of antibacterial agents applied in Danish fish farming. *Archives of Environmental Contamination and Toxicology*, *36*, 1–6.

Martinez, J. L. (2009). Environmental pollution by antibiotics and by antibiotic resistance determinants. *Environmental pollution, 157*, 2893–2902.

Mavronikola, C., Demetriou, M., Hapeshi, E., Partassides, D., Michael, C., Mantzavinos, D. & Kassinos, D. (2009). Mineralisation of the antibiotic amoxicillin in pure and surface waters by artificial UVA- and sunlight-induced Fenton oxidation. *Journal of Chemical Technology Biotechnology*, *84*, 1211–1217.

Minh, T. B., Leung, H. W., Loi, I. H., Chan, W. H., So, M. K., Mao, J. Q., Choi, D., Lam, J. C. W., Zheng, G., Martin, M., Lee, J. H. W., Lam, P. K. S. & Richardson, B. J. (2009). Antibiotics in the Hong Kong metropolitan area: Ubiquitous distribution and fate in Victoria Harbour. *Marine Pollution Bulletin*, *58*, 1052–1062.

Nägele, E. & Moritz, R. (2005). Structure elucidation of degradation products of the antibiotic amoxicillin with ion trap MSn and accurate mass determination by ESI TOF. *Journal of the American Society for Mass Spectrometry*, *16*, 1670–1676.

Official Journal of the European Union, L15/1, Commission Regulation (EU) No 37/2010 of 22 December 2009 on pharmacologically active substances and their classification regarding maximum residue limits in foodstuffs of animal origin, Brussels, Belgium, 2010.

Official Journal of the European Union, L152/11 Regulation (EC) No 470/2009 of the European Parliament and of the Council of 6 May 2009 laying down Community procedures for the establishment of residue limits of pharmacologically active substances in foodstuffs of animal origin, repealing Council Regulation (EEC) No 2377/90 and amending Directive 2001/82/EC of the European Parliament and of the Council and Regulation (EC) No 726/2004 of the European Parliament and of the Council, Strasbourg, France, 2009.

Official Journal of the European Union, L22418, Council Regulation 2377/90/EC of 26 June 1990 laying down a Community procedure for the establishment of maximum residue limits of veterinary medicinal products in foodstuffs of animal origin, Brussels, Belgium, 1990.

Opriş, O., Copaciu, F., Loredana Soran, M., Ristoiu, D., Niinemets, Ü. & Copolovici, L. (2013). Influence of nine antibiotics on key secondary metabolites and physiological characteristics in *Triticum aestivum*: leaf volatiles as a promising new tool to assess toxicity. *Ecotoxicology and Environmental Safety*, *87*, 70–79.

Palmer, P. M., Wilson, L. R., O'Keefe, P., Sheridan, R., King, T. & Chen, C.-Y. (2008). Sources of pharmaceutical pollution in the New York City Watershed. *Science of The Total Environment*, *394*, 90–102.

Pan, X., Deng, C., Zhang, D., Wang, J., Mu, G. & Chen, Y. (2008). Toxic effects of amoxicillin on the photosystem II of *Synechocystis* sp. characterized by a variety of in vivo chlorophyll fluorescence tests. *Aquatic Toxicology*, *89*, 207–213.

Park, S. & Choi, K. (2008). Hazard assessment of commonly used agricultural antibiotics on aquatic ecosystems. *Ecotoxicology*, *17*, 526–538.

Pascoe, D., Karntanut, W. & Müller, C. T. (2003). Do pharmaceuticals affect freshwater invertebrates? A study with the cnidarian *Hydra vulgaris*. *Chemosphere*, *51*, 521–528.

Pérez-Parada, A., Agüera, A., Gómez-Ramos, M. D. M., García-Reyes, J. F., Heinzen, H. & Fernández-Alba, A. R. (2011). Behavior of amoxicillin in wastewater and river water: identification of its main transformation products by liquid chromatography/electrospray quadrupole time-of-flight mass spectrometry. *Rapid Communications in Mass Spectrometry*, *25*, 731–742.

Prescott, J. F. (2007) Beta-lactam Antibiotics: Penam Penicillins. In: Giguere, S., Prescott, J. F., Baggot, J. D., Walker, R. D. & Dowling, P. M. (2007). Antimicrobial Therapy in Veterinary Medicine. *Wiley-Blackwell Publishing,* 4th ed, 121-138.

Ramos, F., Boison, J. & Friedlander, L. G. (2012). "Amoxicillin" in FAO JECFA Monographs 12 – Residue evaluation of certain veterinary drugs. (eds) FAO, Rome – Italy. ISBN 978-92-5-107255-4, 1-35.

Reyns, T., De Boever, S., De Baere, S., De Backer, P. & Croubels, S. (2008). Tissue Depletion of Amoxicillin and Its Major Metabolites in Pigs: Influence of the Administration Route and the Simultaneous Dosage of Clavulanic Acid. *Journal of Agriculture and Food Chemistry*, *56*, 448–454.

Rocca, della, G., Zaghini, A., Zanoni, R., Sanguinetti, V., Zanchetta, S., Di Salvo, A. & Malvisi, J. (2004). Seabream (*Sparus aurata* L.): disposition of amoxicillin after single intravenous or oral administration and multiple dose depletion studies. *Aquaculture*, *232*, 1–10.

Sarmah, A. K., Meyer, M. T. & Boxall, A. B. A. (2006). A global perspective on the use, sales, exposure pathways, occurrence, fate and effects of veterinary antibiotics (VAs) in the environment. *Chemosphere*, *65*, 725–759.

Serrano, P. H. (2005). Responsible Use of Antibiotics Aquaculture, In: FAO Fisheries Technical Paper (FAO), 469 / FAO Rome (Italy) Fishery Industries Div. 97 pp.

Singer, R. S., Finch, R., Wegener, H. C., Bywater, R., Walters, J. & Lipsitch, M. (2003). Antibiotic resistance-the interplay between antibiotic use in animals and human beings. *The Lancet Infectious Diseases*, *3*, 47–51.

Smyth, R. D., Pfeffer, M., Van Harken, D. R., Cohen, A. & Hottendorf, G. H. (1981). Human pharmacokinetics and disposition of sarmoxicillin, a lipophilic amoxicillin prodrug. *Antimicrobial Agents and Chemotherapy*, *19*, 1004–1012.

Tuc Dinh, Q., Alliot, F., Moreau-Guigon, E., Eurin, J., Chevreuil, M. & Labadie, P. (2011). Measurement of trace levels of antibiotics in river water using on-line enrichment and triple-quadrupole LC–MS/MS. *Talanta*, *85*, 1238–1245.

Watkinson, A. J., Murby, E. J. & Costanzo, S. D. (2007). Removal of antibiotics in conventional and advanced wastewater treatment: Implications for environmental discharge and wastewater recycling. *Water Research*, *41*, 4164–4176.

Watkinson, A. J., Murby, E. J., Kolpin, D. W. & Costanzo, S. D. (2009). The occurrence of antibiotics in an urban watershed: From wastewater to drinking water. *Science of The Total Environment*, *407*, 2711–2723.

Zuccato, E., Castiglioni, S., Bagnati, R., Melis, M. & Fanelli, R. (2010). Source, occurrence and fate of antibiotics in the Italian aquatic environment. *Journal of Hazardous Materials*, *179*, 1042–1048.

In: Amoxicillin ISBN: 978-1-62948-489-1
Editors: W. A. Leary and L. M. Kruse

Chapter III

Recent Approaches for the Instrumental Analysis of Amoxicillin

L. K. Bittner, S. A. Schönbichler and C. W. Huck*
Institute of Analytical Chemistry and Radiochemistry,
Leopold-Franzens University, Innsbruck, Austria

1. Abstract

New fast, robust, and accurate instrumental analytical methods for the quality control of the widely-used active pharmaceutical ingredient amoxicillin are of high importance for the pharmaceutical industry. This chapter summarizes recent published new approaches and methods for qualitative and quantitative analysis of amoxicillin and refers to the analysis of other beta-lactam antibiotics. Its main focus is on separation techniques such as high performance liquid chromatography (HPLC) and capillary electrophoresis (CE) and on spectroscopic methods like mid-infrared- (MIR), near-infrared- (NIRS), terahertz- and Raman-spectroscopy. Other focuses are chemiluminescence and UV-vis spectrometric methods, electrochemical methods and paper analytical devices.

* Corresponding Author: christian.w.huck@uibk.ac.at.

2. Introduction

Instrumental analytical methods are of high importance for the quality control in the pharmaceutical industry and replace progressively wet-chemistry methods in pharmacopeias. In the last decades the main focus of research in the field of analytical chemistry was on instrumental analytical methods.

With the launch of the process analytical technology (PAT) initiative [1] by the US-American food and drug administration (FDA) new challenges but also new opportunities for quality control in the pharmaceutical production process opened up. It is of significant importance for manufacturers to guarantee a seamless quality control from incoming raw materials throughout the whole production process till the final product and all of this not only for random samples but for each and every single product. Ideally the production process is monitored on-, at- or in-line. Based on this, vibrational spectroscopic methods became of special interest due to its many advantages such as being non-invasive, fast or cost effective.

Amoxicillin as a well introduced and widespread active pharmaceutical ingredient forms a lead substance when it comes to new analytical methods.

For the analysis of amoxicillin pharmacopeias report chromatography and potentiometric titration methods [2] but there is a remarkable amount of research done to develop new analytical methods for identification and quantification of amoxicillin.

In this chapter the authors summarize new and optimized instrumental analytical methods for the analysis of amoxicillin and other β-lactam antibiotics. It should help the reader to get an overview of what research was done in the last decade about instrumental analysis of amoxicillin.

3. Applications

Capillary Electrophoresis

Santos et al. [3] developed an easy to use and low time consuming method for the simultaneous screening of six antibiotics (ampicillin, amoxicillin, cloxacillin, penicillin, tetracycline and chloramphenicol) in spiked milk samples. They compared Capillary electrophoresis (CE) with high performance liquid chromatography (HPLC) coupled to UV-vis detectors, respectively.

Bailon-Perez and coworkers [4] determined β-lactam antibiotics in waste, well and river water matrices applying capillary zone electrophoresis with UV-diode array detection (CZE-DAD). They used a solvent extraction/solid phase extraction (SPE) method for offline pre-concentration as well as an online pre-concentration method called large volume sample stacking (LVSS) to overcome the low sensitivity of the UV-vis detection.

The same workgroup [5] published a method to determine nine penicillins in environmental water and in chicken muscle using CZE coupled with tandem mass spectrometric detection (CE-MS/MS). Also SPE based pre-concentration and clean up steps are described.

Cruz Oliva et al. [6] reported about a fast CE method to determine bromhexine and amoxicillin in pharmaceutical formulations. UV detection at 214 nm was deployed.

Tian et al. [7] published a CE-method to analyze the penicillin intermediate 6-amino-penicillanic acid and the penicillins penicillin G, ampicillin and amoxicillin in milk.

El-Sabawi and coworkers [8] presented the ability of CE to simplify sample preparation in dissolution testing of amoxicillin. They reported about a CE method to assess the dissolution of amoxicillin in neutral and acidic media in comparison with an official HPLC method.

CE in combination with mass spectrometry (MS) was used for the determination of eight common penicillin antibiotics by Liu et al. [9]. They compared different charged poly(stearyl mathacrylate-divinylbenzene) (poly(SMA-DVB)) monolithic stationary phases. Poly(stearyl mathacrylate-divinylbenzene-vinylbenzyltrimethylammoniumchloride) (poly(SMA-DVB-VBTA)) provided reproducible performance.

Deng et al. [10] published a sensitive method to determine amoxicillin in human urine using CE in combination with electro-chemiluminescence (ECL) detection based on the ECL enhancement of Tris(2,2'-bipyridyl)ruthenium(II) with amoxicillin.

Chemiluminescence and UV-vis Spectrometric Methods

Li et al. [11] presented a flow injection chemiluminescence (CL) method to analyze six different β-lactam antibiotics based on luminol. A possible CL reaction mechanism is discussed.

Jinghua and coworkers [12] developed a flow-injection CL method based on 3-(4'fuorophenyl)-5-(2'sulfonylphenylazo)rhodanine (4FRASP) to determine amoxicillin in capsules.

Sorouraddin et al. [13] established an enhanced thiosemicarbazide(TSC)-H2O2 CL system for the determination of β-lactam antibiotics such as ampicillin sodium and amoxicillin at microgram levels in different pharmaceutical dosage forms.

Hasanpour et al. [14] deployed both, batch and flow injection CL methods to simultaneously analyze the two similar structures of amoxicillin and clavulanic acid. The two chemometric algorithms least squares support vector regression (LS-SVR) and partial least square (PLS) were calculated and compared, with LS-SVR delivering better calibration models.

Jiang and coworkers [15] proposed a method to determine amoxicillin in injections and capsules based on the sensitization effect of cetylpyridine chloride monohydrate (CPC) on the fluorescence of amoxicillin.

Chivulescu et al. [16] analyzed the antibiotics amoxicillin, ampicillin and penicillin using a flow injection analysis method based on CL reaction of β-lactam antibiotics with luminol in basic environment, in presence of ferricyanide and ferrocyanide. This method provided lower detection limits as previous reported similar methods.

Ma and coworkers [17] presented a CL system based on the reaction of Ag(III) complex with luminol in alkaline medium coupled with flow injection analysis to determine penicillin antibiotics in urine and drug samples.

Li et al. [18] described an optimized spectrophotometric method to determine amoxicillin based on the reaction of amoxicillin with 1,2-naphtoquinone-4-sulfonate. The results were compared with official HPLC methods.

Huong and coworkers [19] proposed and compared non-derivative and derivative UV spectrophotometric techniques for the simultaneous determination of amoxicillin and clavulanate in combined tablets. Their results show the applicability for routine analysis.

The workgroup around Gujral [20] presented a UV Spectrophotometric method to determine amoxicillin trihydrate and potassium clavulanate in bulk, pharmaceutical formulation and human urine samples.

Jain et al. [21] quantified amoxicillin trihydrate and ranitidine bismuth simultaneously using UV spectrophotometry.

Jiang et al. [22] studied the color reaction of amoxicillin with victoria blue B resulting in the formation of a red Ion association complex. Based on this reaction a UV spectrophotometric method to analyze amoxicillin was created.

Rojanarata and coworkers [23] developed a fast UV spectrophotometric method for the determination of amoxicillin based on two enzymatic reactions. As all the procedures were performed using no organic solvents and hazardous chemicals and the consumption of chemical is low, this method can be seen as a green analytical method suitable for the quality control of amoxicillin in pharmaceuticals.

Garcia-Reiriz et al. [24] presented the analysis of amoxicillin in human urine by photo-activated generation of fluorescence excitation-emission matrices and artificial neural networks hyphenated with residual bi-linearization.

A real-time optical biosensor method, bio-layer interferometry (BLI), was developed by Scott et al. [25] for the analysis of amoxicillin and other β-lactam antibiotics in water samples.

Electrochemical Methods

Park et al. [26] proposed a potentiometric biosensor system which exploited penicillinase immobilized on Immobilon cellulose nitrate membrane and a pH electrode as the biological component and transducer for screening of penicillin G, amoxicillin and ampicillin.

Zheng and coworkers [27] used the effect that β-cyclodextrin exhibits a pair of reversible peaks in second order differential oscillographic voltagram and the peak height decreases with the concentration increase of an amoxicillin-β-cyclodextrin complex to propose a technique for the analysis of amoxicillin.

Altiokka et al. [28] deployed flow injection analysis with UV detection, potentiometric and conductometric methods to determine amoxicillin in pharmaceuticals.

Kulapina and coworkers [29] presented arrays of potentiometric sensors with plasticized polymer membranes based on tetraalkylammonium organic ion exchangers with anions of penicillin class antibiotics to determine benzyl penicillin, ampicillin, oxacillin and amoxicillin in model mixtures and pharmaceutical preparations.

The same workgroup modified their membranes [30] using silver (I) complexes with ampicillin, oxacillin and cefazolin with tetraalkylammonium organic ion exchangers to quantify antibiotics in model mixtures.

Ensafi et al. [31] deployed multiwall carbon nano tubes decorated with $FeCr_2O_4$ as new electro catalysis for the voltammetric determination of amoxicillin.

Paper Analytical Devices

New fast and easy to handle paper analytical devices are of significant importance for the determination of counterfeit pharmaceuticals, especially in developing countries. They can be a great help for purchasing agents in hospitals [32].

Weaver et al. [33] report about a paper analytical device for fast field screening of β-lactam antibiotics and anti-tuberculosis pharmaceuticals. They developed devices that detect active pharmaceutical ingredients such as ampicillin, amoxicillin, rifampicin, isoniazid, ethambutol and pyrazinamide as well as substitute pharmaceutical such as acetaminophen and chloroquine that may be found in counterfeit pharmaceuticals.

Chromatography, Mass Spectrometry (MS) and Combinations Thereof

Abo El Sooud et al. [34] studied the bioavailability of amoxicillin in chickens after various ways of administration (intravenous, intramuscular and oral). HPLC was deployed to determine the amoxicillin concentrations in plasma.

Averono and coworkers [35] compared orally and intravenous administered amoxicillin/clavulanic acid on patients before tonsillectomy using HPLC methods for the determination of amoxicillin and clavulanic acid in serum and tonsils. Intravenous administration showed better efficacy.

Bogialli et al. [36] developed a fast liquid chromatographic combined with mass spectrometric (LC-MS) method for the determination of amoxicillin and ampicillin in bovine milk, muscle, liver and kidney. This methods shows limits of quantification (LOQ) of <1 ppb in bovine milk.

Idkaidek et al. [37] used HPLC to analyze amoxicillin and clavulanic acid in human plasma for the evaluation of the bioequivalence of two brands of amoxicillin/clavulanic acid combination tablets.

Jensen and coworkers [38] studied the effect of a certain subtype of escherichia coli bacteria on the pharmacokinetics of orally administered amoxicillin in piglets using HPLC for quantitative analysis of amoxicillin in plasma.

Letendre and coworkers [39] deployed LC-MS/MS as a tool to determine amoxicillin, antipyrine, atenolol, propranolol and testosterone in plasma to evaluate the roles of gastrointestinal absorption and hepatic extraction as barriers to oral bioavailability.

Yoon et al. [40] developed a HPLC-MS method for simultaneous determination of amoxicillin and clavulanic acid in human plasma using terbutaline as internal standard. Very low LOQs could be achieved (0,12 μg/mL for amoxicillin and 0,062 μg/mL for clavulanic acid).

Dousa et al. [41] proposed a HPLC method for routine identification and quantification of amoxicillin in premixes.

Du and coworkers [42] published a HPLC technique for the analysis of amoxicillin in mouse serum and broncho-alveolar lavage (BAL) fluid.

Karlage et al. [43] studied the content uniformity and weight variation for three pharmaceutical products (amoxicillin, amoxicillin/clavulanic acid and furosemide) bought in pharmacies in the United States and Mexico using HPLC as an analytical tool.

Liu et al. [44] published an ion exchange HPLC method for the simultaneous determination of flucloxacillin and amoxicillin in pharmaceutical formulations for injection.

A method for quantification for tracing the amount of penicillin contaminants in an active pharmaceutical ingredient (API) based on HPLC-MS was proposed by Takada and coworkers [45].

Tattevin et al. [46] published a work how to apply HPLC to monitor β-lactam antibiotics plasma concentrations during the treatment of endocarditis.

AlGaai and coworkers [47] utilized HPLC to measure amoxicillin concentration in deproteinized serum to study the bioequivalence of two amoxicillin formulations.

Li and coworkers [48] developed a HPLC method with UV detection at 230 nm for the simultaneous determination of amoxicillin and ranitidine in rat plasma.

Perez-Lozano et al. [49] described a methodology to monitor amoxicillin and degradation products during a stability evaluation in a solid premix veterinary formulation applying reversed phase HPLC.

Amoxicillin in surplus plasma of neonates using reversed phase HPLC was determined by Pullen et al. [50] to study pharmacokinetics and dosing of amoxicillin in (pre)term neonates.

Samanidou and coworkers [51] presented the development and validation of a HPLC method to determine amoxicillin, oxacillin, cloxacillin and dicloxacillin in human biological fluids.

The workgroup around Baglie [52] deployed HPLC and HPLC electron spray ionization MS (HPLC-ESI-MS) to analyze plasma and salivary amoxicillin concentrations.

Cavazos-Rocha et al. [53] reported about HPLC methods with UV and fluorescence detection to investigate five different antimicrobials (amoxicillin, trimethoprim, linezolid, sulfamethoxazole and garenoxacin) in plasma and tissue of actinomycetoma.

De Baere et al. [54] published a HPLC-MS/MS method to quantify amoxicillin in animal feed.

A technique to determine amoxicillin and clavulanic acid in human plasma using isocratic reverse phase HPLC in combination with UV detection was proposed by Foroutan et al. [55].

Godejohann et al. [56] used hydrophilic interaction chromatography in combination with nuclear magnetic resonance spectroscopy and MS to separate and identify the endogenous metabolite trigonelline and the polar antibiotic amoxicillin in human urine.

Gonzalez-San Miguel and coworkers [57] developed a technique based on multi-syringe chromatography to analyze amoxicillin, ampicillin and cephalexin.

Pullen et al. [58] published a reversed phase HPLC assays in combination with UV detection for the determination of amoxicillin and rifampicin in neonatal plasma.

A simple, sensitive and robust reversed phase HPLC method was developed and validated by Tavakoli et al. [59] for the simultaneous determination of amoxicillin and metronidazole using the single wavelength of 254 nm.

Xu and coworkers [60] analyzed antibiotics in the Victoria Harbor and the Pearl River in southern China using HPLC-ESI-MS.

Grujic at al. [61] studied the formation of the protonated methanol-adduct of amoxicillin using HPLC coupled to ESI-MS.

Khuroo and coworkers [62] worked on an optimized HPLC-MS method for the determination of amoxicillin in human plasma.

Kyricos and coworkers [63] evaluated the quality of amoxicillin formulations in in Egypt, Jordan, Lebanon and Saudi Arabia using HPLC.

Mastovska and coworkers [64] developed an HPLC-MS method for the multiresidue analysis of β-lactam antibiotics in bovine kidneys.

Muller et al. [65, 66] deployed HPLC assays for the study of pharmacokinetics of amoxicillin in pregnant women.

Reyns et al. [67-69] presented a fast method for the quantitative determination of amoxicillin, amoxicilloic acid and amoxicillin diketopiperazine-2', 5'-dione in kidney, liver, fat and muscle of pigs based on HPLC-ESI-MS/MS and studied the tissue depletion of amoxicillin and its major metabolites.

Teixeira and coworkers [70] developed a screening procedure for antibiotics in waste water by direct HPLC analysis with UV detection.

Wen et al. [71] developed and validated a LC-MS/MS method for the determination of amoxicillin and ambroxol in human plasma and applied this technique for pharmacokinetic studies.

Beltran and coworkers [72] described a cephalexin molecularly imprinted polymer for solid phase extraction with liquid chromatography to analyze cephalexin and amoxicillin in urine.

Benito-Pena [73] published a method to quantify penicillin V and amoxicillin in feed samples applying HPLC with UV detection.

Braun et al. [74] used HPLC to quantify amoxicillin in bovine uterine tissue.

Del Tacca et al. [75] utilized HPLC to study the bioequivalence between generic and branded amoxicillin formulations in a clinical study.

Längin and coworkers [76] studied the transformation of the two β-lactam antibiotic amoxicillin and piperacillin in biodegradability tests applying HPLC with UV detection and HPLC-MS/MS as analytical tools.

Nikam et al. [77] developed and validated a reversed phase HPLC method for the simultaneous estimation of amoxicillin trihydrate and flucloxacillin sodium in capsules.

Ortelli and coworkers [78] published an ultra-performance LC coupled to time of flight (TOF)-MS technique for a fast multiresidue screening of 150 veterinary drugs in milk.

Linear gradient HPLC, utilized for the analysis of amoxicillin and related substances, was described by Raju et al. [79].

Shukla et al [80] deployed HPLC for the quantification and prediction of skin pharmacokinetics of amoxicillin and cefuroxime.

HPLC with UV detection was deployed by Averono et al. [81] to determine amoxicillin concentration in plasma and tissue in pediatric patients undergoing tonsillectomy.

Boscher et al. [82] developed a method for the quantification of 33 veterinary drug residues in feeding stuffs by HPLC-MS.

Dhoka and coworkers [83] presented a high performance thin layer chromatographic (HPTLC) method to determine amoxicillin trihydrate and bromhexine hydrochloride in oral solid dosage forms.

Hoang Vu et al. [84] compared reverse phase HPLC and UV spectrophotometric methods for the simultaneous determination of amoxicillin and cloxacillin in capsules and suggested the interchangeability between these two methods for the routine analysis.

Jayakar et al. [85] developed and validated a reversed phase HPLC method for the simultaneous determination of amoxicillin and potassium clavulanate.

Sonawane and coworkers [86] published a reversed phase HPLC method for the simultaneous determination of amoxicillin trihydrate and bromhexine hydrochloride from oily suspensions.

Tippa et al. [87] proposed a validated HPLC method to analyze amoxicillin and clavulanic acid in injections.

Zheng et al. [88] utilized an HPLC method to study transfer and distribution of amoxicillin in plasma, gastric mucosa and gastric juice of rats.

Buszewski et al. [89] presented an approach to determine amoxicillin in human plasma using solid phase micro extraction based on conducting polymers in combination with HPLC.

Chitlange and coworkers [90] proposed two methods for the simultaneous quantitative analysis of amoxicillin trihydrate and ambroxol hydrochloride based on UV spectroscopy and reversed phase HPLC. Both methods show correlation coefficients of nearly 1.

Dinh et al. [91] presented a technique to measure trace levels of antibiotics in river water using on-line enrichment and LC-MS/MS.

Idris et al. [92] compared sequential injection chromatography with HPLC and CE. The sequential injection chromatographic method has shown some advantages over HPLC and CE analysis with respect to reagent consumption and sample frequency.

Kaufmann and coworkers [93] developed an improved high resolution mass spectrometry based multi-residue method for veterinary drugs in different food matrices using a single stage orbit trap mass spectrometer.

An analytical method based on ultra-high performance liquid chromatography (UHPLC) with tandem mass spectrometry for the simultaneous determination of amoxicillin, penicillin G and their major metabolites was published by Liu et al. [94]

Lugoboni et al. [95] developed and validated a LC-MS/MS method for the quantitative analysis of amoxicillin in bovine muscle.

Pei and coworkers [96] worked on a HPLC-DAD method to determine amoxicillin and sulbacatam in human plasma for bioequivalence studies.

Verdier et al. [97] described a HPLC method with UV detection for the simultaneous determination of twelve β-lactam antibiotics (amoxicillin, cefepime, cefotaxime, ceftazidime, ceftriaxone, cloxacillin, imipenem, meropenem, oxacillin, penicillin G, piperacillin and ticarcillin) which could be used in routine therapeutic drug monitoring.

Beg et al. [98] report about a reversed phase HPLC method to quantify amoxicillin trihydrate in pharmaceutical formulations and bulk using box-behnken experimental design. The experimental design was validated employing analysis of variance (ANOVA) calculation.

A HPLC method for the simultaneous estimation of amoxicillin trihydrate and tinidazole is described by Bojaraju and coworkers [99].

Dong et al. [100] reports about an LC-MS/MS method operated in segmental and multiple reaction monitoring for the simultaneous determination of amoxicillin and ambroxol in human plasma. The method was employed for a pharmacokinetic study of amoxicillin and ambroxol hydrochloride tablets.

Kowalczuk et al. [101] presented a HPLC with UV detection method for the analysis of amoxicillin after pre-column derivatization of amoxicillin with 1-[(quinolin-6-ylcarbamoyl)oxy]pyrrolidine-2,5-dione (AccQ-Fluor).

Li and coworkers [102] developed a UHPLC method tandem MS for the simultaneous determination of amoxicillin and prednisolone in bovine milk.

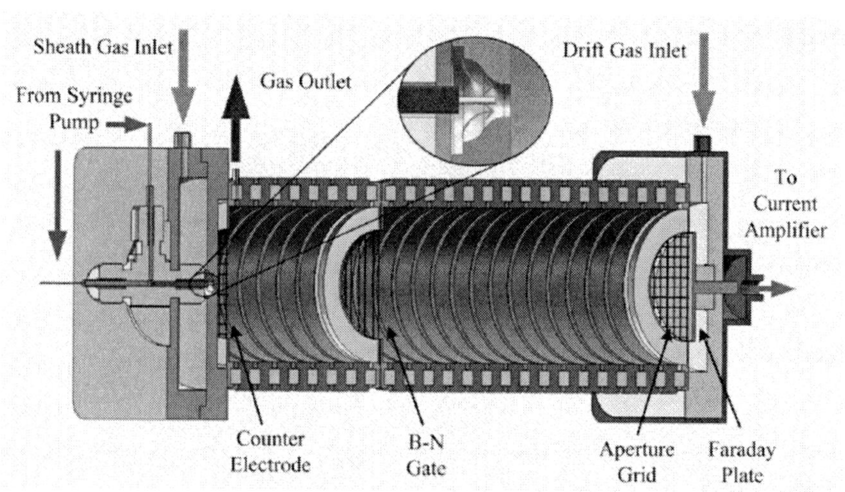

Figure 1. Scheme of an ESI-IMS system. Reproduced with permission from [103].

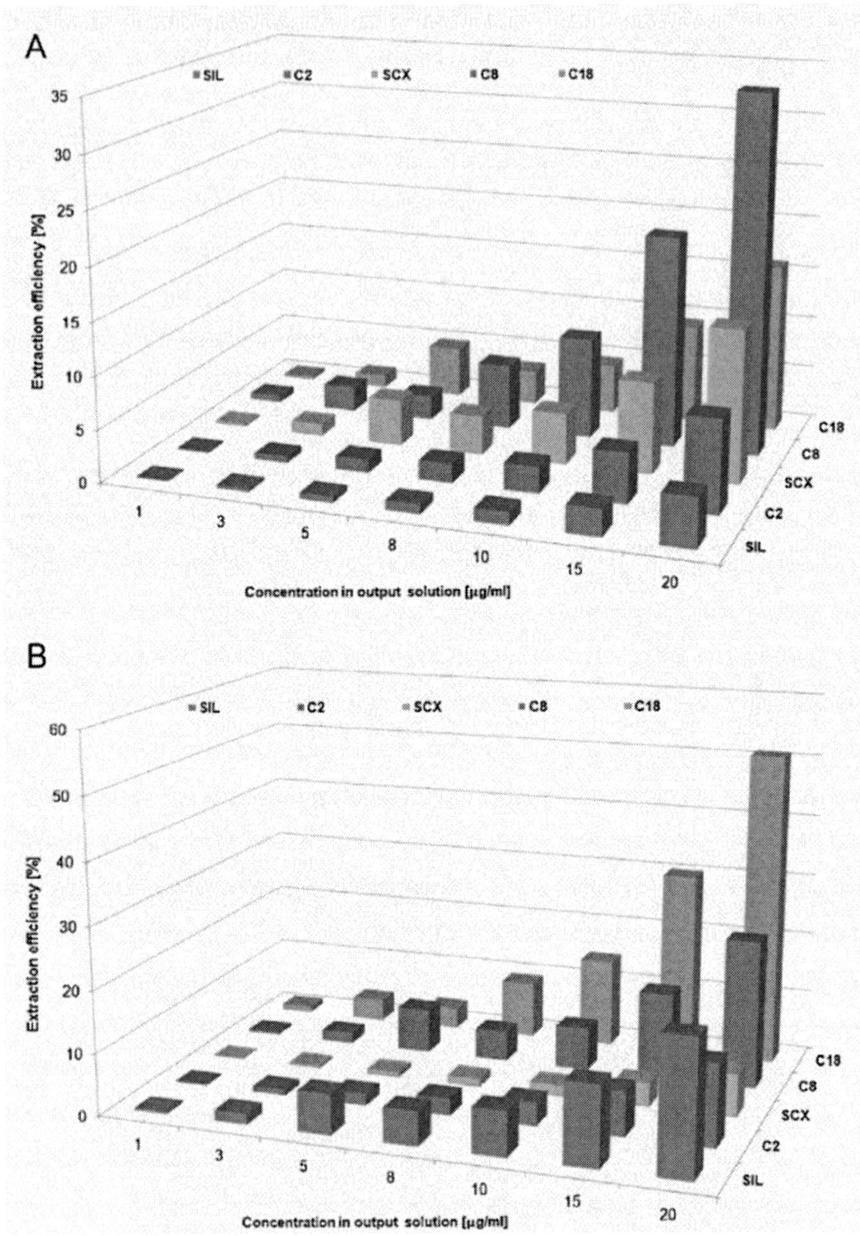

Figure 2. Comparison of the performance of five different MEPS sorbents for (A) linezolid and (B) amoxicillin extracted from human plasma. Reproduced with permission from [105].

Li et al. [103] proved the feasibility of using electrospray ionization ion mobility spectrometry (ESI-IMS) to analyze antibiotics in liquid samples. Figure 1 shows the scheme of an ESI-IMS system.

Macarov and coworkers [104] developed a multiresidue analysis to determine the content of penicillins regulated by the European Union in bovine, porcine and chicken muscle using LC-MS/MS.

Szultka et al. [105] developed and compared LC-MS methods to determine linezolid and amoxicillin in human plasma. Samples were prepared applying protein precipitation, solid phase extraction and micro extraction in packed syringes (MEPS). Figure 2 presents the performances of different MEPS.

The same workgroup reported the development of molecular imprinted solid phase micro extraction fibers and the application for antibiotic drugs by SPME-LC/MS [106].

Xi et al. [107] presented a HPLC tandem MS method for the simultaneous determination of amoxicillin and clavulanic acid in dog plasma. The method was utilized for pharmacokinetic studies of the above mentioned active pharmaceutical ingredients in healthy beagles.

Xie and coworkers [108] proposed a method for the simultaneous analysis of amoxicillin and ampicillin in eggs using HPLC with fluorescence detection after pre-column derivatization.

Xu et al. [109] established a HPLC-MS/MS method for the determination of amoxicillin in honey.

Berendsen at al. [110] utilized HPLC coupled to tandem mass spectrometry for the analysis of amoxicillin and other β-lactam antibiotics in poultry muscle.

Dong et al. [111] developed a sample preparation method for measuring amoxicillin in human plasma by hollow fiber centrifugal ultrafiltration (HF-CF-UF) prior to HPLC analysis.

Mid-infrared-, Near-infrared-, Terahertz- and Raman Spectroscopic Methods

Müller et al. [112] developed a method for the simultaneous determination of clavulanic acid and amoxicillin in tablets using diffuse reflectance infrared fourier transform spectroscopy (DRIFTS) and multivariate calibration. Calibration models were established using PLS, interval PLS and synergy interval PLS algorithms.

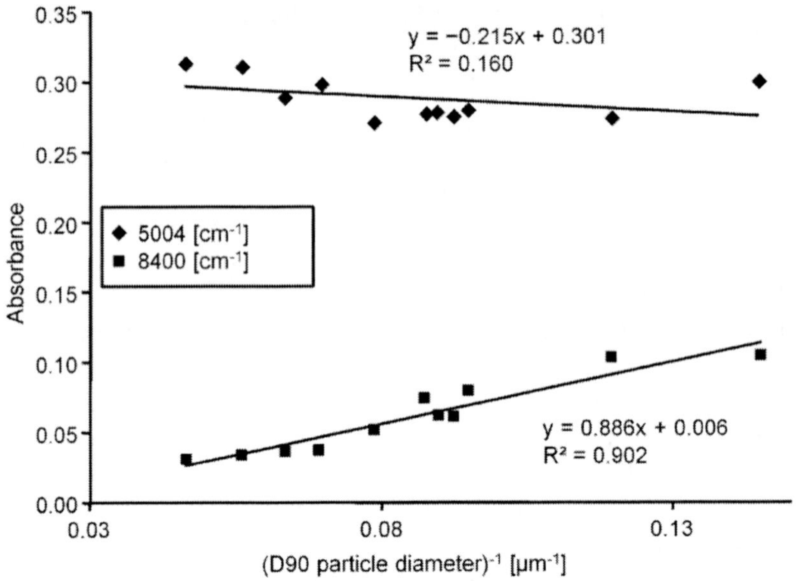

Figure 3. Correlation between absorbance and reciprocal D90 particle diameter at specific wavenumbers. Reproduced with permission from [114].

Qu and coworkers [113] deployed near infrared spectroscopy (NIRS) in combination with multivariate data analysis and artificial neural networks (ANN) for the analysis of amoxicillin in powder.

Bittner et al. [114] developed a method based on NIRS in diffuse reflection mode for the simultaneous identification and particle size determination of amoxicillin bulk powder. A correlation between absorbance and reciprocal D90 particle diameter at specific wavenumbers was observed and is shown in figure 3.

In a recent publication Silva and coworkers [115] developed and validated a multivariate calibration method for the determination of amoxicillin in suspension formulations by NIRS.

Terahertz time-domain spectroscopy was utilized by Li et al. [116] to investigate amoxicillin capsules. They showed that this relative new technique could be a powerful tool for quality control in the pharmaceutical industry.

Chen et al. [117] proposed a terahertz spectroscopic quantitative method using an adaptive micro-genetic algorithm with a variable internal population to analyze mixtures of methamphetamine, heroin and amoxicillin.

Meng and coworkers [118] set up a terahertz time-domain system to detect amoxicillin medicines.

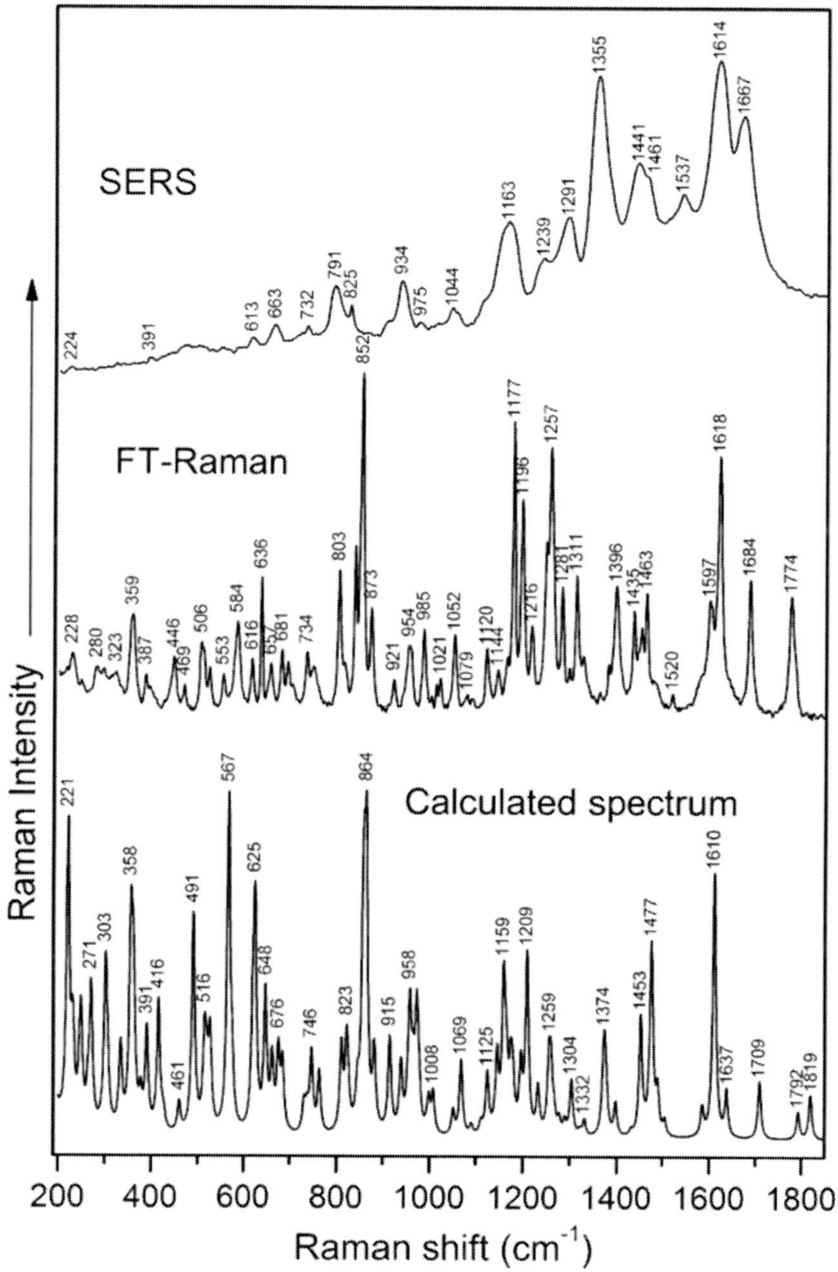

Figure 4. Comparison of the SERS- and the Raman-spectra with the DFT calculated spectrum. Reproduced with permission from [120].

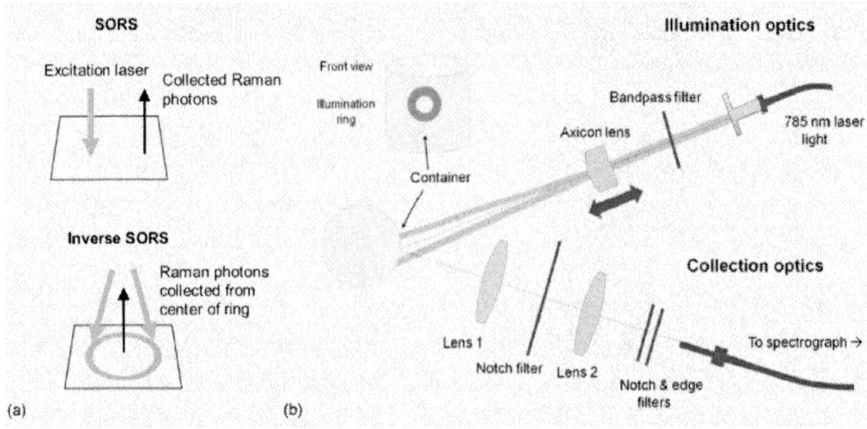

Figure 5. (a) Schematic diagram of SORS and inverse SORS. (b) Inverse SORS instrument design. Reproduced with permission from [121].

Bugay and coworkers [119] studied the possibilities of handheld Raman spectrometers to identify various widespread pharmaceutical active ingredients. They present a novel decision algorithm for the assessment of the correlation between the Raman spectrum of the unknown sample and the spectrum of the reference material.

Bebu et al. [120] report about a study of amoxicillin using IR, Raman, surface enhanced Raman spectroscopy (SERS) and chemical calculations based on density functional theory (DFT). Figure 4 compares the SERS- and the Raman-spectra with the DFT calculated spectrum.

Olds and coworkers [121] deployed spatially offset Raman spectroscopy (SORS) for the analysis and detection of packaged pharmaceuticals and concealed drugs. Figure 5 illustrates the principle of SORS and inverse SORS.

Ji et al. [122] developed a SERS method for the analysis of amoxicillin residues in foods.

4. Perspective

In recent years a growing number of reports about new methods and procedures for the identification and quantification of amoxicillin and other β-lactam antibiotics were published. Whilst still HPLC based techniques are the majority reported, there is an increase of new methods such as spectroscopic methods (mid-IR, NIR, terahertz spectroscopy or Raman spectroscopy) which can be observed over the last years. This can be of significant interest for the pharmaceutical industry especially regarding process analytical technology (PAT).

References

[1] K. A. Bakeev, Process analytical technology: spectroscopic tools and implementation strategies for the chemical and pharmaceutical industries. Wiley.com, (2010).

[2] S. P. Kaur, R. Rao and S. Nanda, *Int. J. Pharm. Pharm. Sci.* 3, 30-37 (2011).

[3] S. M. Santos, M. Henriques, A. C. Duarte and V.I. Esteves, Talanta 71, 731-737 (2007).

[4] M. Bailón-Pérez, A. Garcia-Campana, C. Cruces-Blanco and M. del Olmo Iruela, *J. Chromatogr.* A 1185, 273-280 (2008).

[5] I. M. Bailón-Pérez, A. M. García-Campaña, M. del Olmo Iruela, C. Cruces-Blanco and L. G. Gracia, *Electrophoresis* 30, 1708-1717 (2009).

[6] D. Cruz Oliva, K. Torres Vélez and A. L. Revilla Vázquez, *Journal of the Mexican Chemical Society* 55, 79-83 (2011).

[7] C. Tian, H. Tan, L. Gao, H. Shen and K. Qi, *Chinese journal of chromatography* 29, 1128 (2011).

[8] D. El-Sabawi, I. I. Hamdan and D. Haj-Ali, *J. Liq. Chromatogr. Relat. Technol.* 35, 573-589 (2012).

[9] W.-L. Liu, C.-Y. Wu and H.-Y. Huang, *Talanta* (2012).

[10] B. Deng, A. Shi, L. Li and Y. Kang, *J. Pharm. Biomed. Anal.* 48, 1249-1253 (2008).

[11] Y. Li and J. Lu, *Luminescence* 21, 251-255 (2006).

[12] Y. Jinghua, W. Fu-Wei, D. Ping, H. Jiadong and C. Jian-Jie. Determination of Amoxicillin with Novel Rhodanine Ramification by Flow Injection Chemiluminescence. in Bioinformatics and Biomedical Engineering, 2009. ICBBE 2009. 3rd International Conference on. 2009: IEEE.

[13] M. Sorouraddin, M. Iranifam and A. Imani-Nabiyyi, *Luminescence* 24, 102-107 (2009).

[14] F. Hasanpour, A. A. Ensafi and T. Khayamian, *Anal. Chim. Acta* 670, 44-50 (2010).

[15] H. Jiang, M. Feng and H. Zhang, Physical Testing and Chemical Analysis (Part B: Chemical Analysis) 12, 035 (2010).
[16] A. I. Chivulescu, M. Badea-Doni, M.-C. Cheregi and A. F. Danet, *Rev. Roum. Chim.* 56, 247-254 (2011).
[17] L. Ma, W. Jun Kang, X. Dong Xu, L. Mei Niu, H. Mei Shi and S. Li, *J. Anal. Chem.* 67, 219-225 (2012).
[18] Q. Li and Z. Yang, *Anal. Lett.* 39, 763-775 (2006).
[19] V. T. Huong and V. D. Hoang, *Int. J. Pharm. Tech. Res.* 1, 1173-1181 (2009).
[20] R. S. Gujral and S. M. Haque, *International journal of biomedical science* 6, 335 (2010).
[21] A. K. Jain, N. Lariya, A. Agarwal, A. K. Kharya and G. P. Agrawal, *Int. J. Chem. Res.* 1, 41-5 (2010).
[22] H. Jiang, H. Zhang and H. Xie, *Chemical Research and Application* 4, 016 (2010).
[23] T. Rojanarata, P. Opanasopit, T. Ngawhirunpat, C. Saehuan, S. Wiyakrutta and V. Meevootisom, *Enzyme Microb. Technol.* 46, 292-296 (2010).
[24] A. Garcia-Reiriz, P. C. Damiani and A. C. Olivieri, *Anal. Chim. Acta* 588, 192-9 (2007).
[25] I. M. Scott, L. J. Kraft, J. D. Parker, K. Daniel, S. Kustick, D. Kennen, J.L. McMurry and J. L. McMurry, Academy of Science 68, 72 (2010).
[26] I.-S. Park, D.-K. Kim and N. Kim, *J. Microbiol. Biotechnol.* 14, 698-706 (2004).
[27] J. Zheng and F. Tao, *Chinese Journal of Applied Chemistry* 22, 599 (2005).
[28] G. Altiokka, N.Ö. Can and H.Y. Aboul-Enein, *J. Liq. Chromatogr. Relat. Technol.* 30, 1333-1341 (2007).
[29] E. Kulapina, S. Snesarev, N. Makarova and E. Pogorelova, *J. Anal. Chem.* 66, 78-83 (2011).
[30] E. Kulapina and S. Snesarev, *J. Anal. Chem.* 67, 163-167 (2012).
[31] A. A. Ensafi, A. R. Allafchian and B. Rezaei, *Journal of Nanoparticle Research* 14, 1-11 (2012).
[32] C. H. Arnaud, *Chem. Eng. News* 90, 30-34 (2012).
[33] A. A. Weaver, H. Reiser, T. L. Barstis, M. Benvenuti, D. Ghosh, M. Hunckler, B. Joy, L. Koenig, K. Raddell and M. Lieberman, *Anal. Chem.* (2013).
[34] K. Abo El-Sooud, Y. H. Al-Tarazi and M. M. Al-Bataineh, *Vet. Res. Commun.* 28, 599-607 (2004).

[35] G. Averono, M. Olina, M. Basile, M. Bagnati, A. Uglietti, P. L. Garavelli, G. Bellomo and F. Pia, *Recenti Prog. Med.* 95, 314-5 (2004).
[36] S. Bogialli, V. Capitolino, R. Curini, A. Di Corcia, M. Nazzari and M. Sergi, *J. Agric. Food Chem.* 52, 3286-91 (2004).
[37] N.M. Idkaidek, A. Al-Ghazawi and N.M. Najib, Biopharm. Drug Dispos. 25, 367-72 (2004).
[38] G. M. Jensen, J. Lykkesfeldt, K. Frydendahl, K. Moller and O. Svendsen, *Am. J. Vet. Res.* 65, 992-5 (2004).
[39] L. Letendre, M. Scott, G. Dobson, I. Hidalgo and B. Aungst, *Pharm. Res.* 21, 1457-62 (2004).
[40] K. H. Yoon, S. Y. Lee, W. Kim, J. S. Park and H. J. Kim, *J. Chromatogr. B Analyt. Technol. Biomed. Life. Sci.* 813, 121-7 (2004).
[41] M. Dousa and R. Hosmanova, *J. Pharm. Biomed. Anal.* 37, 373-7 (2005).
[42] X. Du, C. Li, H. K. Sun, C. H. Nightingale and D. P. Nicolau, *J. Pharm. Biomed. Anal.* 39, 648-52 (2005).
[43] K. L. Karlage and P. B. Myrdal, *Drug Dev. Ind. Pharm.* 31, 993-1000 (2005).
[44] H. Liu, H. Wang and V. B. Sunderland, *J. Pharm. Biomed. Anal.* 37, 395-8 (2005).
[45] W. Takada, T. Adachi, N. Kihara, S. Kitamura, T. Kitagawa, M. Mifune and Y. Saito, *Chem. Pharm. Bull.* (Tokyo) 53, 172-6 (2005).
[46] P. Tattevin, O. Tribut, C. Arvieux, M. Dupont, R. Flicoteaux, L. Desbordes, Y. Le Tulzo and C. Michelet, *Clin. Microbiol. Infect.* 11, 76-9 (2005).
[47] E. AlGaai, S. AlDigither, M. Lockyer and M. M. Hammami, *Arzneimittelforschung*. 56, 48-51 (2006).
[48] W. Li, F. Tan and K. Zhao, *J. Pharm. Biomed. Anal.* 41, 594-8 (2006).
[49] P. Perez-Lozano, E. Garcia-Montoya, A. Orriols, M. Minarro, J. R. Tico and J. M. Sune-Negre, *J. Pharm. Biomed. Anal.* 42, 192-9 (2006).
[50] J. Pullen, L. M. Stolk, F. H. Nieman, P. L. Degraeuwe, F. H. van Tiel and L. J. Zimmermann, *Ther. Drug Monit.* 28, 226-31 (2006).
[51] V. F. Samanidou, E. N. Evaggelopoulou and I. N. Papadoyannis, *J. Sep. Sci.* 29, 1550-60 (2006).
[52] S. Baglie, A. P. Del Ruenis, R. H. Motta, R. C. Baglie, G. C. Franco, L. M. Franco, P. L. Rosalen, P. Silva and F. C. Groppo, *Int. J. Clin. Pharmacol. Ther.* 45, 556-62 (2007).

[53] N. Cavazos-Rocha, L. Vera-Cabrera, O. Welsh-Lozano, N. Waksman-de-Torres and M. de la Luz Salazar-Cavazos, *J. Pharm. Biomed. Anal.* 43, 1775-81 (2007).

[54] S. De Baere and P. De Backer, *Anal. Chim. Acta* 586, 319-25 (2007).

[55] S. M. Foroutan, A. Zarghi, A. Shafaati, A. Khoddam and H. Movahed, *J. Pharm. Biomed. Anal.* 45, 531-4 (2007).

[56] M. Godejohann, *J. Chromatogr.* A 1156, 87-93 (2007).

[57] H. M. Gonzalez-San Miguel, J. M. Alpizar-Lorenzo and V. Cerda, *Anal. Bioanal. Chem.* 387, 663-71 (2007).

[58] J. Pullen, L. M. Stolk, C. Neef and L. J. Zimmermann, *Biomed. Chromatogr.* 21, 1259-65 (2007).

[59] N. Tavakoli, J. Varshosaz, F. Dorkoosh and M. R. Zargarzadeh, *J. Pharm. Biomed. Anal.* 43, 325-9 (2007).

[60] W. H. Xu, G. Zhang, S. C. Zou, X. D. Li and Y. C. Liu, *Environ. Pollut.* 145, 672-9 (2007).

[61] S. Grujic, T. Vasiljevic, M. Lausevic and T. Ast, *Rapid Commun. Mass Spectrom.* 22, 67-74 (2008).

[62] A. H. Khuroo, T. Monif, P. R. Verma and S. Gurule, *J. Chromatogr. Sci.* 46, 854-61 (2008).

[63] S. Kyriacos, M. Mroueh, R. P. Chahine and O. Khouzam, *J. Clin. Pharm. Ther.* 33, 375-9 (2008).

[64] K. Mastovska and A. R. Lightfield, *J. Chromatogr.* A 1202, 118-23 (2008).

[65] A. E. Muller, J. DeJongh, P. M. Oostvogel, R. A. Voskuyl, P. J. Dorr, M. Danhof and J. W. Mouton, *Am. J. Obstet. Gynecol.* 198, 108 e1-6 (2008).

[66] A. E. Muller, P. J. Dorr, J. W. Mouton, J. De Jongh, P. M. Oostvogel, E. A. Steegers, R. A. Voskuyl and M. Danhof, *Br. J. Clin. Pharmacol.* 66, 866-74 (2008).

[67] T. Reyns, M. Cherlet, S. De Baere, P. De Backer and S. Croubels, *J. Chromatogr. B Analyt. Technol. Biomed. Life. Sci.* 861, 108-16 (2008).

[68] T. Reyns, S. De Boever, S. De Baere, P. De Backer and S. Croubels, J. *Agric. Food Chem.* 56, 448-54 (2008).

[69] T. Reyns, S. De Boever, S. Schauvliege, F. Gasthuys, G. Meissonnier, I. Oswald, P. De Backer and S. Croubels, *J. Vet. Pharmacol. Ther.* 32, 241-8 (2009).

[70] S. Teixeira, C. Delerue-Matos, A. Alves and L. Santos, *J. Sep. Sci.* 31, 2924-31 (2008).

[71] A. Wen, T. Hang, S. Chen, Z. Wang, L. Ding, Y. Tian, M. Zhang and X. Xu, *J. Pharm. Biomed. Anal.* 48, 829-34 (2008).
[72] A. Beltran, N. Fontanals, R. M. Marce, P. A. Cormack and F. Borrull, *J. Sep. Sci.* 32, 3319-26 (2009).
[73] E. Benito-Pena, J. L. Urraca and M. C. Moreno-Bondi, *J. Pharm. Biomed. Anal.* 49, 289-94 (2009).
[74] M. Braun, H. Zerbe and M. Kietzmann, *Berl. Munch. Tierarztl. Wochenschr.* 122, 51-7 (2009).
[75] M. Del Tacca, G. Pasqualetti, A. Di Paolo, A. Virdis, G. Massimetti, G. Gori, D. Versari, S. Taddei and C. Blandizzi, *Br. J. Clin. Pharmacol.* 68, 34-42 (2009).
[76] A. Langin, R. Alexy, A. Konig and K. Kummerer, *Chemosphere* 75, 347-54 (2009).
[77] D.S. Nikam, C.G. Bonde, S. Surana, G. Venkateshwarlu and P. Dekate, *Inter. J. of Pharm.Tech. Res.* 1, 935-939 (2009).
[78] D. Ortelli, E. Cognard, P. Jan and P. Edder, *J. Chromatogr.* B 877, 2363-2374 (2009).
[79] C.B. Raju, H. Sharma, C.S. Rao and G. Rao, *Acta Chromatographica* 21, 57-70 (2009).
[80] C. Shukla, V. Patel, R. Juluru and G. Stagni, *Biopharm. Drug Dispos.* 30, 281-93 (2009).
[81] G. Averono, M. Vidali, M. Olina, M. Basile, M. Bagnati, G. Bellomo and P. Aluffi, *Int. J. Pediatr. Otorhinolaryngol.* 74, 995-8 (2010).
[82] A. Boscher, C. Guignard, T. Pellet, L. Hoffmann and T. Bohn, *J. Chromatogr.* A 1217, 6394-6404 (2010).
[83] M. Dhoka, V. Gawande and P. Joshi, *J. Pharma. Sci. Res.* 2, 477-483 (2010).
[84] D. Hoang Vu and T. Giang Do, *Journal of Young Pharmacists* 2, 190-195 (2010).
[85] B. Jayakar, M. Kumar, M. Kumudhavalli and C. Saravanan, *Int. J. Pharm. Tech. Res.* 2, 906-9 (2010).
[86] L. Sonawane and S. Bari, *Pharm. Anal. Acta* 1, 2153-2435 (2010).
[87] D. M. R. Tippa and N. Singh, *American Journal of Analytical Chemistry* 1, 95-101 (2010).
[88] H. L. Zheng, Y. M. Hu, J. J. Bao and J. M. Xu, *Acta Pharmacol. Sin.* 31, 501-8 (2010).
[89] B. Buszewski, M. Szultka, P. Olszowy, S. Bocian and T. Ligor, *Analyst* 136, 2635-42 (2011).

[90] S. S. Chitlange, S. R. Tawargeri and K.K. Chaturvedi, *Asian Journal of Research in Chemistry* 4, 1025-1030 (2011).

[91] Q. T. Dinh, F. Alliot, E. Moreau-Guigon, J. Eurin, M. Chevreuil and P. Labadie, *Talanta* 85, 1238-45 (2011).

[92] A. M. Idris and R. E. Elgorashe, *Microchem. J.* 99, 174-179 (2011).

[93] A. Kaufmann, P. Butcher, K. Maden, S. Walker and M. Widmer, *Anal. Chim. Acta* 700, 86-94 (2011).

[94] C. Liu, H. Wang, Y. Jiang and Z. Du, *J. Chromatogr. B Analyt. Technol. Biomed. Life. Sci.* 879, 533-40 (2011).

[95] B. Lugoboni, T. Gazzotti, E. Zironi, A. Barbarossa and G. Pagliuca, *J. Chromatogr. B Analyt. Technol. Biomed. Life. Sci.* 879, 1980-6 (2011).

[96] Q. Pei, G.P. Yang, Z. J. Li, X. D. Peng, J. H. Fan and Z. Q. Liu, *J. Chromatogr. B Analyt. Technol. Biomed. Life. Sci.* 879, 2000-4 (2011).

[97] M.-C. Verdier, O. Tribut, P. Tattevin, Y. Le Tulzo, C. Michelet and D. Bentué-Ferrer, *Antimicrob. Agents Chemother.* (2011).

[98] S. Beg, K. Kohli, S. Swain and M. S. Hasnain, *J. Liq. Chromatogr. Relat. Technol.* 35, 393-406 (2012).

[99] V. Bojaraju, D. Sireesha, V. Prasad and P. V. Diwan, *World Journal of Chemistry* 7, 47-52 (2012).

[100] X. Dong, L. Ding, X. Cao, L. Jiang and S. Zhong, *Biomed. Chromatogr.* (2012).

[101] D. Kowalczuk and A. Galewska, *Pol. J. Environ. Stud.* 21, 139-143 (2012).

[102] H. Li, X. Xia, Y. Xue, S. Tang, X. Xiao, J. Li and J. Shen, *J. Chromatogr. B Analyt. Technol. Biomed. Life. Sci.* 900, 59-63 (2012).

[103] S. Li, J. Jia, X. Gao, X. He and J. Li, *Anal. Chim. Acta* 720, 97-103 (2012).

[104] C. Macarov, L. Tong, M. Martínez-Huélamo, M. Hermo, E. Chirila, Y. Wang, D. Barrón and J. Barbosa, *Food Chem.* (2012).

[105] M. Szultka, R. Krzeminski, J. Szeliga, M. Jackowski and B. Buszewski, *J. Chromatogr.* A (2012).

[106] M. Szultka, J. Szeliga, M. Jackowski and B. Buszewski, *Anal. Bioanal. Chem.* 403, 785-96 (2012).

[107] W. Xi, L. He, C. Guo, Q. Cai and Z. Zeng, *Anal. Lett.* 45, 1764-1776 (2012).

[108] K. Xie, L. Jia, D. Xu, H. Guo, X. Xie, Y. Huang, X. Chen, W. Bao, G. Dai and J. Wang, *J. Chromatogr. Sci.* 50, 620-4 (2012).

[109] W. Xu, X. Zhang, B. Wu, Y. Yin, W. Yang, C. Shen, T. Ding and H. Chen, *Chinese journal of chromatography* 30, 1089-1092 (2012).

[110] B. J. Berendsen, H. W. Gerritsen, R. S. Wegh, S. Lameris, R. van Sebille, A. A. Stolker and M. W. Nielen, *Anal. Bioanal. Chem.* 1-16 (2013).
[111] W. C. Dong, Z. L. Hou, X. H. Jiang and Y. Jiang, *J. Chromatogr. Sci.* 51, 181-6 (2013).
[112] A. L. Muller, R. S. Picoloto, M. F. Ferrao, F. E. da Silva, E. I. Muller and E. M. Flores, *Drug testing and analysis* 4, 500-6 (2012).
[113] N. Qu, M. Zhu, H. Mi, Y. Dou and Y. Ren, Spectrochim. *Acta. A. Mol. Biomol. Spectrosc.* 70, 1146-51 (2008).
[114] L. K. Bittner, N. Heigl, C. H. Petter, M. F. Noisternig, U. J. Griesser, G. K. Bonn and C. W. Huck, *J. Pharm. Biomed. Anal.* 54, 1059-64 (2011).
[115] M. A. Silva, M. H. Ferreira, J. W. Braga and M. M. Sena, *Talanta* 89, 342-51 (2012).
[116] N. Li, J. Shen, Y. Jia and C. Zhang, *Spectrosc. Spectral Anal.* 27, 1692 (2007).
[117] Y. Chen, Y. Ma, Z. Lu, B. Peng and Q. Chen, *J. Appl. Phys.* 110, 044902 (2011).
[118] K. Meng, Z. Li and Q. Liu. The detection of amoxicillin medicines by terahertz time-domain spectroscopy. in Photonics and Optoelectronics Meetings 2011. 2012: International Society for Optics and Photonics.
[119] D. E. Bugay and R. C. Brush, *Appl. Spectrosc.* 64, 467-475 (2010).
[120] A. Bebu, L. Szabó, N. Leopold, C. Berindean and L. David, *J. Mol. Struct.* 993, 52-56 (2011).
[121] W. J. Olds, E. Jaatinen, P. Fredericks, B. Cletus, H. Panayiotou and E. L. Izake, *Forensic Sci. Int.* 212, 69-77 (2011).
[122] W. Ji, H. Qian and W. Yao, *Spectrosc. Lett.* (2013).

In: Amoxicillin ISBN: 978-1-62948-489-1
Editors: W. A. Leary and L. M. Kruse

Chapter IV

Amoxicillin: Pharmaceutical Properties and Clinical Applications

Nico T. Mutters, M.D., M.P.H.[1,*]
and Eva Meyle, R.Ph.[2]
[1]Department of Infectious Diseases, Heidelberg University Hospital, Heidelberg, Germany
[2]Department of Pharmacy, Heidelberg University Hospital, Heidelberg, Germany

Abstract

Amoxicillin represents the lead substance of the aminopenicillin group of beta-lactams, which is characterized by a broader antibacterial spectrum and acid-stability compared to penicillin G. It is the hydroxylated derivative of ampicillin and is used orally because of its nearly full oral bioavailability and its high tissue diffusion, however, it has a short terminal half-life of only 1 - 1.5 hours.

Amoxicillin is a very popular antibiotic, especially by family practitioners. In 2010, amoxicillin was the fifth most commonly

* E-mail: nico.mutters@med.uni-heidelberg.de.Phone: +49-6221-5636289. Fax: +49-6221-565857.

prescribed generic medication of the USA. Like for all other beta-lactams its bactericidal activity is based on the inhibition of the bacterial cell wall synthesis by inactivating enzymes, so-called penicillin binding proteins, which are located in the cell membrane. Amoxicillin is active against a broad spectrum of Gram-positive (not *S. aureus*, not *E. faecium*) and Gram-negative (not *P. aeruginosa*, *Enterobacter spp*., *Klebsiella spp.* etc.) bacteria, however, it has no activity against anaerobic bacteria.

In the last decades the emergence and spread of β-lactamases has become a major problem for the medical use of Amoxicillin. The β-lactamases - including plasmid-mediated AmpC enzymes, extended-spectrum β-lactamases (ESBL) and carbapenemases – mediate resistance to different or all classes of beta-lactams. Nevertheless, the medical use of amoxicillin still is various. Especially in infections of the ENT area it is commonly used and well proven for the empiric treatment of otitis media, sinusitis, tonsillitis, and pharyngitis. However, it is also indicated for non-severe respiratory infections such as community-acquired pneumonia as well as for uncomplicated urinary tract infections in woman. Furthermore, oral amoxicillin administration is recommended by national and international guidelines for prophylaxis of infective endocarditis, especially for the treatment of infective endocarditis due to enterococci or oral streptococci.

Amoxicillin is generally considered a well-tolerated drug; however, there are several potential adverse effects and contraindications the physician has to take in mind. The most important contraindication is a known allergy or hypersensitivity against penicillin's or any other beta-lactams. The administration of amoxicillin to a patient with a history of beta-lactam hypersensitivity can lead to severe anaphylactic reactions which sometimes can be fatal. Other adverse events are occurrence of gastrointestinal symptoms, such as diarrhoea, or exanthema (on average 8%). Especially in patients with infectious mononucleosis, other viral diseases, or lymphocytic leukemia exanthema is significantly more frequent.

Mechanism of Action

Amoxicillin belongs to the beta-lactam group of antibacterials. It is a semi synthetic, acid-stable penicillin with moderate antibacterial spectrum covering a wide range of Gram-positive and a limited range of Gram-negative bacteria. Since it was introduced in the early 1970s [1], it is still of great importance for the therapy of various different infections today.

Together amoxicillin and ampicillin form the group of aminopenicillins, the name derived from their special chemical structure that distinguishes these beta-lactam antibiotics from others (Figure 1). Their identical antibacterial spectrum and close pharmacological relationship can be explained by a slight difference in their chemical structure.

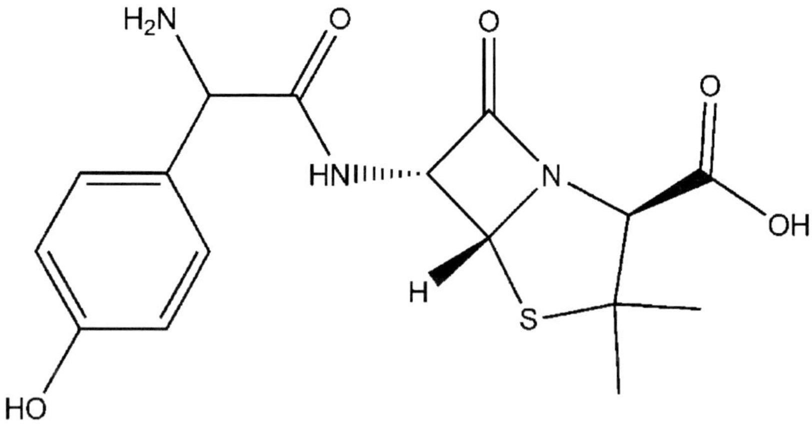

Figure 1. Amoxicillin.

Amoxicillin is the p-hydroxylated derivative of ampicillin, the pioneer aminopenicillin. Although not differing in antimicrobial potency the structural modification of adding a hydroxyl group changes the physicochemical properties of ampicillin. That also accounts for pharmacokinetic differences between ampicillin and amoxicillin.

The antibacterial action is based on the inhibition of the bacterial cell wall synthesis by a mechanism which is well known for all penicillins and other beta-lactam antibiotics (cephalosporins, carbapenems and monobactams). Amoxicillin binds to a bacterial transpeptidase, called penicillin-binding protein (PBP) 1A. PBPs constitute a group of enzymes involved in cross-linking two linear peptidoglycan-chains. The PBPs are transmembrane proteins; their active site is localized on the outside of the cell-membrane. Thereby PBP's assist the last step of cell wall synthesis. By opening the amoxicillin's lactam-ring the C-terminal transpeptidase-domain gets irreversibly acylated. Disturbance of bacterial cell-wall synthesis integrity by amoxicillin leads to bacterial cell lysis resulting in a bactericidal effect [2, 3].

As mentioned above the slight chemical difference compared to ampicillin does not change the antibacterial spectrum or the potency [4]. Amoxicillin was from the beginning of its use a potent antibacterial drug, however, associated with an important problem all penicillins were confronted with at that time: The susceptibility to beta-lactamases, enzymes, conferring penicillin-resistance to the bacteria by destroying the beta-lactam ring before binding to their target site. To avoid irreversible destruction by beta-lactamases amoxicillin is often administered in fixed combinations with clavulanic acid, a beta-lactamase inhibitor (Figure 2).

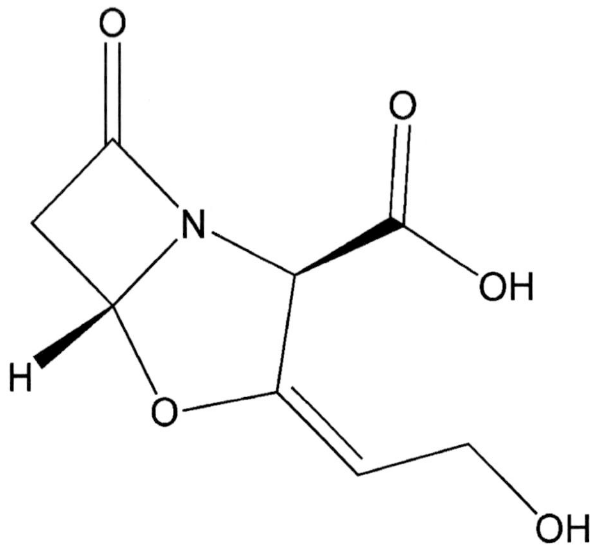

Figure 2.Clavulanic acid.

Clavulanic acid is a natural product of *Streptococcus clavuligerus* and was discovered in 1972. Although structurally related to penicillins it has only low antibacterial potency but a higher affinity to the beta-lactamase compared to the antibacterial compound amoxicillin. By binding to the beta-lactamase the enzyme gets irreversibly inhibited [5-7].

Pharmacokinetics and –Dynamics (PK/PD)

Amoxicillin is acid-stable and can be taken orally without being irreversibly hydrolyzed by gastric acid. Additionally, parenteral formulations for intravenous or intramuscular application are available as well. Oral administered amoxicillin is nearly completely absorbed. Concomitant food intake does not change the degree of absorption, so that peak serum concentrations are attained within 1 to 2 hours after administration. Compared to ampicillin the exposition of amoxicillin is 2 to 2.5 times higher than that achieved by oral ampicillin. Approximately 17-20% of the dose is blood-protein bound and the distribution volume is about 0.3-0.4 L/kg. During the rapid distribution phase tissue penetration reaches mostly all human body fluids and bones, except of the eyes and normal meninges. Amoxicillin will reach effective antibacterial concentrations in ascitic fluid, synovial fluid, bone tissues, gynecological tissues, sputum and, what is important for the pediatric population, in middle-ear fluid. Even in state of acute inflammation with a meningeal penetration rate of up to 80%, penetration in cerebrospinal fluid, however, is still considered sub-optimal [8, 9]. Amoxicillin has a short terminal half-life of only 0.7-1.4 hours in adults with normal renal function indicating that there is no accumulation following rapid administration of multiple doses.

Amoxicillin undergoes partial metabolism in the liver resulting in microbiologically inactive metabolites. Approximately 60% of the dose is eliminated in the urine in unchanged form and only small amounts are excreted in bile and feces. Latest pharmacokinetic studies in critically ill patients evolved that pharmacokinetic parameters vary widely in this collective, however, dosage adjustment is not recommended if renal function is normal [10].

Regarding the amoxicillin/clavulanic acid combination similar serum profiles are expected due to similar pharmacokinetic behavior of the two substances.

Commonly amoxicillin is taken orally. As oral formulations, capsules, coated tablets or dispersible tablets are available; all of them contain the trihydrate form of amoxicillin. In addition, oral formulation for pediatric patients is provided as solid powder which can be mixed with drinking water giving a suspension. Intravenous (I.V.) infusion is uncommon but some manufacturers provide powder for intravenous use after dissolution. For treating mild infections adult dosage is 500-1000mg orally every 8 or 12 hours respectively.

In cases of more severe infections dosage can be raised to 1g every 6hours. Pediatric dosage range is between 50 and 100 mg/KG body weight per day divided in two to three doses [11]. Dosage regimen for the combination of amoxicillin/clavulanic acid is normally 875mg/125mg orally b.i.d.. In cases of more severe infections I.V. administration is recommended in higher doses ranging between 1000mg amoxicillin/ 200mg clavulanic acid or 2000/ 200mg as single dose [12]. Maximum daily dose of amoxicillin is 6000mg. Dose reduction is recommended in patients with severe renal failure. If glomerular filtration rate (GFR) is 10ml/min to 30ml/min the oral dosage should be reduced to 250mg or 500mg every 12 hours and in patients with GFR below 10ml/min dosage interval should be increased to 24 hours. In patients undergoing intermittent hemodialysis maintenance dose should be 0.5-1g and administration on hemodialysis days should take place after dialysis. If continuous ambulant peritoneal dialysis is applied 0.5-1g amoxicillin should be given on dialysis days. Frequency of dosing should be raised to 12 hours in patients under continuous venovenous hemofiltration or hemodialysis [13].

Regarding the PK/PD relationship amoxicillin, like other penicillins, exhibits time-dependent killing type. That means that the T>MIC is the parameter that correlates best with its efficacy. For sufficient antibiotic efficacy the established target value for T>MIC is 40% [14]. At concentrations 3- to 4-fold higher than the MIC maximum killing is achieved and above this concentration no additional killing effect can be detected [15-17]. Amoxicillin produces a short post-antibacterial effect of 1.5-2 hours, which has been shown for staphylococci and streptococci [18, 19].

Potential Adverse Effects

Amoxicillin is commonly well tolerated. The most frequently reported side effects are gastrointestinal disturbances like diarrhea (4-15%), nausea and vomiting (3-6%) [20-22]. Common adverse events are due to immunologic reactions, mostly affecting the skin. Allergic reactions to beta-lactams occur in 0.7-8% of treated patients. Whereas typical Type-I-reactions with skin rashes, urticaria or purpura are uncommon and angio-edema or even life-threatening anaphylaxis are rare, a more common skin reaction is the so-called “fifth day rash” expressed as a maculopapular or mobilliform exanthema.

The former hypersensitivity reactions are also called immediate because they arise ~1h after drug intake and are IgE-mediated. In contrary the latter ones are T-cell-mediated and called non-immediate, occurring delayed (later than 1h after intake) and even after the end of the therapy. Of importance is the fact that about 30% of children co-infected with Eppstein-Barr-Virus show non-immediate skin reactions when treated with Amoxicillin [23]. There have been a few cases of toxic epidermal necrolysis and Stevens-Johnson-Syndrome described, however, this is considered a very rare event [24]. The risk of severe skin-reactions is more often associated with amoxicillin/clavulanic acid-combination therapy than with amoxicillin alone. Regarding cross-reactivity among penicillins and the structural related cephalosporins, carbapenems and monobactams data suggest a rate between 0.17-8.4% of the patients who report penicillin reactions will react if given a cephalosporin [25-30]. For carbapenems the rate of cross-reactivity of skin-test proven penicillin-IgE-mediated allergic patients has shown to be at 1% [31-34]. Among antibiotics amoxicillin/clavulanic acid is the one most frequent associated with liver injury, as well as the most frequently prescribed drug leading to hospitalization for drug-induced liver disease [35-40]. The occurrence of liver-injury starts days to weeks after the beginning of treatment and is typically characterized by cholestatic hepatitis. These data, however, could be attributed to the fact that Amoxicillin is very popular and often prescribed in the out-patient setting promoting the high incidence of adverse events.

Although transient elevation of serum transaminases is not uncommon after amoxicillin and amoxicillin/clavulanic acid therapy, hepatic injuries are rare [36, 41].

Amoxicillin alone shows a significant lower incidence of liver injuries, counting for a direct involvement of clavulanic acid in the pathogenesis of these adverse effects. From all patients 0.1-1% suffer from headache or dizziness during therapy with amoxicillin. Changes of the blood cell count, resulting in a clinical picture of reversible leukopenia, agranulocytosis or prolongation of prothrombin time occur very rarely [24]. In addition, adverse renal effects might occur after amoxicillin administration, however, it is rare and probably not dose related [42].

Drug-Drug-Interactions

As mentioned above Amoxicillin is a well-tolerated substance and there are only few things to consider when combined with other drugs. Like all antibacterial substances amoxicillin can disturb the gut flora leading to lower systemic exposure of hormones from oral contraceptives or impairing the enterohepatic circulation of mycophenolic acid. Due to active tubular secretion elimination half-life is increased by concomitant use of probenecid. Concurrent administration can lead to increased and prolonged blood levels of amoxicillin. Further patients receiving amoxicillin and oral anticoagulants have to be monitored appropriately for prolongation of prothrombin time (increased international normalized ratio). Disturbance of the gut flora might lead to decreased systemic vitamin K levels [43, 44]. Co-therapy with allopurinol could increase the risk of developing rashes as adverse events.

Pregnancy and Breast Feeding

Amoxicillin, like other penicillins, is a drug of choice for treating infections with sensible organisms during pregnancy and is categorized as B according to the United States Food and Drug Administration's Risk Category (all trimesters). There is no proven increase in the frequency of malformations or harmful effects on the fetus and animal studies do not indicate a risk [45]. Amoxicillin is also considered compatible with breastfeeding. The milk to maternal plasma ratio ranges between 0.013-0.05 [46], and only 0.7% of adult dose could be detected in breast milk [47].

Medical Use

Amoxicillin is a very popular antibiotic, especially by family practitioners and pediatricians. In 2010, amoxicillin was the fifth most commonly prescribed generic medication of the USA. Amoxicillin is active against a broad spectrum of Gram-positive (not *S. aureus*, not *E. faecium*) and Gram-negative (not *P. aeruginosa*, *Enterobacter spp.*, *Klebsiella spp.* etc.) bacteria, however, it has no activity against anaerobic bacteria. It can be combined with the beta-lactamase inhibitor clavulanic acid to reach a broader activity spectrum, including Gram-positive (not *E. faecium*) and Gram-negative bacteria particularly *H. influenzae*, beta-lactamase forming pathogens and anaerobes.

Due to its broad spectrum activity and the nearly complete absorption after oral administration, amoxicillin is well suited for outpatient use and treatment of mild infections. Especially for infections of the Ear-Nose-Throat (ENT) area, it is commonly used and well proven for the empiric treatment of acute otitis media, sinusitis, tonsillitis, and pharyngitis.

A recent study from North America, however, stated that due to the distribution of bacteria causing acute otitis media amoxicillin/clavulanate in high dosage would be the preferred treatment over amoxicillin alone [48]. The influence of the pneumococcal conjugate vaccination and antibiotic selection pressure has resulted in a predominance of beta-lactamase-producing *Haemophilus influenzae* followed by penicillin-resistant *Streptococcus pneumonia* [48]. This distribution, however, depends most likely on the local epidemiology and on local vaccination rates. According to the results of the SAUCE 4 study, for instance, the pneumococcal resistances to penicillin in Spain have fallen drastically [49, 50]. Since *Streptococcus pneumoniae* is the bacterial agent which is the most common bacteria in acute otitis media [49], amoxicillin would still be the appropriate and the by guidelines endorsed drug of choice. Acute otitis media is very common in infants and small children and often symptoms are rather general than specific; thus, acute otitis media should be considered in any child with unexplained diarrhea, vomiting or fever. If the infection is inadequately treated, there may be chronic infection and discharge through a perforated drum, accompanied by impaired hearing. Amoxicillin is also recommended for the empirical treatment of acute sinusitis. While pathogenesis and etiology are analogous to those of acute otitis media, symptoms may be localized tenderness, facial pain and fever. Identification of the causative bacteria is possible by culture of pus aspirate from the sinus; however, often treatment is administered without microbiological diagnostics.

In case of more severe infections in the ENT area, such as mastoiditis, odontogenic abscesses, sinusitis with orbital involvement or neck phlegmons, treatment should be initiated with parenteral amoxicillin/clavulanate, because of the regular involvement of beta-lactamase-producing bacteria and anaerobes.

Another application for amoxicillin is for respiratory tract infections. Although the respiratory tract is without interruption from nose to lungs, it is common to distinguish between infections of the upper and lower respiratory tract. In case of lower respiratory tract infections the two main important types of infections are bronchitis and pneumonia. The causative agents of infectious acute bronchitis are mainly viruses; however, secondary bacterial infections do also play a role in the pathogenesis. Antibiotic treatment may therefore be indicated, however, a microbiological diagnosis should be made.

Pneumonia, on the other hand, is the most common cause of infection-related death in Europe and the USA. The causative agents are manifold and symptoms are not specific per pathogen. While the clinical diagnosis of pneumonia may often be easy, the identification of the microbial cause is often challenging. In young children, however, in whom bacterial and viral infections can occur with similar frequencies, clinical diagnosis of pneumonia may be more challenging [51].

The infection occurs via inhalation of aerosolized material or aspiration. Dependent on the size of inhaled particles they are able to reach the alveoli. Infections can occur in healthy individuals due to pathogens possessing adhesins and other virulence factors to attach to and infiltrate the respiratory tract. In addition, immunocompromised patients may develop infections with microorganisms that do not infect healthy individuals. Based on pathological and radiologic findings, four terms have been established to classify pneumonia: lobar pneumonia, bronchopneumonia, necrotizing pneumonia, and interstitial pneumonia. Another rather clinical classification defines pneumonia based on the place of acquisition: Community-acquired pneumonia (CAP), hospital-acquired (nosocomial) pneumonia (HAP), and healthcare-associated pneumonia (HCAP), which is acquired in other healthcare facilities, such as long-term healthcare facilities or nursing homes. For the treatment of CAP in children, which have been appropriately immunized, amoxicillin (90mg/kg/d orally in 2 doses) is recommended as first-line therapy for presumed bacterial pneumonia [51, 52]. In addition, for non-severe cases of CAP in adults, amoxicillin is also recommended as first choice for treatment [49, 53, 54]. In case of HCAP and HAP, however, microbiological diagnosis should accompany empirical treatment since the frequency of resistant pathogens and beta-lactamase producing pathogens is much higher than in the outpatient setting.

Besides the use of amoxicillin in pulmonology it is equally important in cardiology; especially in the context of infective endocarditis. Infective endocarditis is a disease which often presents as fever of unknown origin and if left untreated, can be fatal. It can be rapidly progressive as well as subacute. Most of the patients suffering of infective endocarditis have pre-existing heart defects which had made them more susceptible to infectious agents. Native valves are usually infected by oral streptococci (viridans group) while coagulase-negative staphylococci are more common in prosthetic valve endocarditis. In principle, any bacteremia can cause infective endocarditis. It is therefore of main importance to prevent bacteremia in patients with pre-existing heart defects to minimize the risk of infection. Especially since the mortality of infective endocarditis is high (20-50%) despite antibiotic treatment.

Oral amoxicillin administration is thus recommended by national and international guidelines for prophylaxis of infective endocarditis [55]. It should be administered to patients with pre-existing heart defects when bacteremia is likely to occur, for example during dental procedures. Amoxicillin, possibly in combination with gentamicin is also recommended for the treatment of infective endocarditis due to enterococci and oral streptococci [55].

Amoxicillin is sometimes recommended for the treatment of mastitis in breastfeeding woman. There is, however, insufficient evidence to confirm or refute the effectiveness of antibiotic therapy for the treatment of lactational mastitis [56].

Antimicrobial Resistance

In the last decades the emergence and spread of beta-lactamases has become a major problem for the medical use of amoxicillin. The beta-lactamases - including plasmid-mediated AmpC enzymes, extended-spectrum beta-lactamases (ESBL), and carbapenemases – mediate resistance to different or all classes of beta-lactams. In the early 1980s third-generation cephalosporins were introduced into clinical practice and considered a major breakthrough in the fight against beta-lactamase-mediated bacterial resistance to antibiotics [57]. They had been developed in response to the increased prevalence of beta-lactamases in certain organisms (for example, ampicillin hydrolyzing TEM-1 in *Escherichia coli*) and the spread of these beta-lactamases into new hosts (for example, *Haemophilus influenzae*) [57]. It did not take long, however, until the first plasmid encoded beta-lactamases occurred that were able to hydrolyze the new developed cephalosporins [58]. These and other soon discovered beta-lactamases were summarized and called ESBLs. Besides beta-lactamases other resistance mechanisms such as increased expression of efflux systems or reduced porin expression have been described [59, 60]. These mechanism, however, are mainly contributory factors while spread of ESBLs and carbapenemases is considered the greater threat. These enzymes are released into the periplasmic space and hydrolyze the beta-lactams before they can reach their target structure, the PBPs. The first in *E. coli* discovered plasmid-encoded beta-lactamase TEM-1, mediating resistance to ampicillin and cephalotin, probably derived from the chromosomally encoded SHV-1 from *Klebsiella pneumonia* [61]. Meanwhile, hundred types of TEM and SHV have been described [62]. In the fight against the increasing resistance, especially among Gram-negatives, beta-lactamase inhibitors such as clavulanic acid were initially developed and combinations such as amoxicillin/clavulanate were successfully used. However, even simple amino acid substitutions caused by point mutations can lead to changes in the binding sites of the catalytic centre rendering the beta-lactamase inhibitors useless. Another strategy is the overexpression of beta-lactamases so that after all inhibitors have bound, there are still sufficient beta-lactamases available to hydrolyze the beta-lactam antibiotic. Nowadays overwhelming numbers and classes of beta-lactamases have been described. The CTX-M group, the OXA-beta-lactamases (e.g. OXA-48), AmpC, and the metallo-beta-lactamases, such as VIM and IMP to only name a few. The main issue is the transferability of many of those beta-lactamases between different bacterial species. In response to that threat different surveillance systems were launched. For example, the European Antimicrobial Resistance Surveillance System (EARSS) in which more than 30 European countries participate. The Centers for Disease Control and Prevention (CDC) in the USA launched numerous surveillance systems that collect data on antibiotic/antimicrobial resistance and drug susceptibility, as well. Surveillance is the first step of infection control and provides the ability to identify increasing incidences of infections with multidrug-resistant gram-negatives (MDR-GN) and to take action against it. Infections with MDR-GN result in longer inpatient stays and higher costs compared with those with nonresistant gram-negative organisms and are associated with a high mortality and morbidity [63, 64]. As antibiotic treatment of MDR-GN is extremely difficult the need for development of new antibiotics is pressing; this development, however, is very hesitant. When today's antibiotics such as amoxicillin have no effect due to spreading resistance among bacteria, new antibiotics will be critically necessary to save lives.

Acknowledgments

The authors declare that they have no conflict of interests.

References

[1] Sabto J., Carson P., Morgan T. Evaluation of amoxycillin--a new semisynthetic penicillin. *Med. J. Aust.,* 1973;2(11):537-41.

[2] Neu H. C. Penicillins--new insights into their mechanisms of activity and clinical use. *Bull. N Y Acad. Med.,* 1982;58(8):681-95.

[3] Zervosen A., Sauvage E., Frere J. M., Charlier P., Luxen A. Development of new drugs for an old target: the penicillin binding proteins. *Molecules,*17(11):12478-505.

[4] Brogden R. N., Heel R. C., Speight T. M., Avery G. S. Amoxycillin injectable: a review of its antibacterial spectrum, pharmacokinetics and therapeutic use. *Drugs,* 1979;18(3):169-84.

[5] Rolinson G. N. 6-APA and the development of the beta-lactam antibiotics. *J.Antimicrob.Chemother.,* 1979;5(1):7-14.

[6] White A. R., Kaye C., Poupard J., Pypstra R., Woodnutt G., Wynne B. Augmentin (amoxicillin/clavulanate) in the treatment of community-acquired respiratory tract infection: a review of the continuing development of an innovative antimicrobial agent. *J.Antimicrob.Chemother.,* 2004;53 Suppl 1:i3-20.

[7] Reading C., Cole M. Clavulanic acid: a beta-lactamase-inhiting beta-lactam from Streptomyces clavuligerus. *Antimicrob. Agents Chemother.,*1977;11(5):852-7.

[8] Bakken J. S., Bruun J. N., Gaustad P., Tasker T. C. Penetration of amoxicillin and potassium clavulanate into the cerebrospinal fluid of patients with inflamed meninges. *Antimicrob. Agents Chemother.,* 1986;30(3):481-4.

[9] Decazes J. M., Bure A., Wolff M., Kitzis M. D., Pangon B., Modai J. Bactericidal activity against Haemophilusinfluenzae of cerebrospinal fluid of patients given amoxicillin-clavulanic acid. *Antimicrob. Agents Chemother.,* 1987;31(12):2018-9.

[10] Carlier M., Noe M., De Waele J. J., Stove V., Verstraete A. G., Lipman J. et al. Population pharmacokinetics and dosing simulations of amoxicillin/clavulanic acid in critically ill patients. *J.Antimicrob.Chemother.*, 2013.

[11] GlaxoSmithKlineUK. Summary of product characteristics: Amoxil® vials for injection 1g. Middlesex, UK: GlaxoSmithKlineUK; 2012.

[12] GlaxoSmithKlineUK. Summary of product characteristics: Augmentin® intravenous. Dublin, Ireland2013.

[13] Frank U., Tacconlli E. The Daschner Guide to In-Hospital Antibiotic Therapy 2012-2013. 2 ed. Heidelberg: Springer; 2012.

[14] Sanchez Navarro A. New formulations of amoxicillin/clavulanic acid: a pharmacokinetic and pharmacodynamic review. *Clin.Pharmacokinet.,* 2005;44(11):1097-115.

[15] Turnidge J. D. The pharmacodynamics of beta-lactams. *Clin. Infect. Dis.*, 1998;27(1):10-22.

[16] Hyatt J. M., McKinnon P. S., Zimmer G. S., Schentag J. J. The importance of pharmacokinetic/pharmacodynamic surrogate markers to outcome. Focus on antibacterial agents. *Clin.Pharmacokinet.,* 1995;28(2):143-60.

[17] Mouton J. W., Vinks A. A. Is continuous infusion of beta-lactam antibiotics worthwhile?--efficacy and pharmacokinetic considerations. *J.Antimicrob.Chemother.*, 1996;38(1):5-15.

[18] Craig W., Gudmundsson S. The postantibiotic effect. In: Lorian V, editor. Antibiotics in laboratory medicine. 2 ed. Baltimore (MD): William and Wilkins; 1986. p. 515-63.

[19] Thorburn C. E., Molesworth S. J., Sutherland R., Rittenhouse S. Postantibiotic and post-beta-lactamase inhibitor effects of amoxicillin plus clavulanate. *Antimicrob. Agents Chemother.*, 1996;40(12):2796-801.

[20] Neu H. C., Wilson A. P., Gruneberg R. N. Amoxycillin/clavulanic acid: a review of its efficacy in over 38,500 patients from 1979 to 1992. *J.Chemother.,* 1993;5(2):67-93.

[21] Martinez-Mir I., Ferrer J. M., Palop V., Estan L., Rubio E., Morales-Olivas F. J. Are the adverse drug reactions of amoxycillin and amoxycillin-clavulanic acid similar? *Pharmacoepidemiol. Drug Saf.,* 1996;5(4):247-54.

[22] Salvo F., Polimeni G., Moretti U., Conforti A., Leone R., Leoni O. et al. Adverse drug reactions related to amoxicillin alone and in association with clavulanic acid: data from spontaneous reporting in Italy. *J.Antimicrob.Chemother.*, 2007;60(1):121-6.

[23] Chovel-Sella A., Ben Tov A., Lahav E., Mor O., Rudich H., Paret G. et al. Incidence of rash after amoxicillin treatment in children with infectious mononucleosis. *Pediatrics,* 2012;131(5):e1424-7.

[24] Kaur S. P., Rao R., Nanda S. Amoxicillin: a broad spectrum antibiotic. International *Journal of Pharmacy and Pharmaceutical Sciences,* 2011;3(3):30-7.

[25] Petz L. D. Immunologic cross-reactivity between penicillins and cephalosporins: a review. *J. Infect. Dis.,* 1978;137 Suppl:S74-S9.

[26] Dash C. H. Penicillin allergy and the cephalosporins. *J.Antimicrob.Chemother.,* 1975;1(3 Suppl):107-18.

[27] Daulat S., Solensky R., Earl H. S., Casey W., Gruchalla R. S. Safety of cephalosporin administration to patients with histories of penicillin allergy. *J. Allergy Clin.Immunol.,* 2004;113(6):1220-2.

[28] Goodman E. J., Morgan M. J., Johnson P. A., Nichols B. A., Denk N., Gold B. B. Cephalosporins can be given to penicillin-allergic patients who do not exhibit an anaphylactic response. *J.Clin.Anesth.*, 2001;13(8):561-4.

[29] Fonacier L., Hirschberg R., Gerson S. Adverse drug reactions to acephalosporins in hospitalized patients with a history of penicillin allergy. *Allergy Asthma Proc.*, 2005;26(2):135-41.

[30] Pederson-Bjergaard J. Cephalothin in the treatment pf penicillin sensitive patients. *Acta.Allergol.,* 1967;22:299.

[31] Atanaskovic-Markovic M., Gaeta F., Medjo B., Viola M., Nestorovic B., Romano A. Tolerability of meropenem in children with IgE-mediated hypersensitivity to penicillins. *Allergy,* 2008;63(2):237-40.

[32] Romano A., Viola M., Gueant-Rodriguez R. M., Gaeta F., Valluzzi R., Gueant J. L. Brief communication: tolerability of meropenem in patients with IgE-mediated hypersensitivity to penicillins. *Ann. Intern. Med.,* 2007;146(4):266-9.

[33] Romano A., Viola M., Gueant-Rodriguez R. M., Gaeta F., Pettinato R., Gueant J. L. Imipenem in patients with immediate hypersensitivity to penicillins. *N. Engl. J. Med.,* 2006;354(26):2835-7.

[34] Atanaskovic-Markovic M., Gaeta F., Gavrovic-Jankulovic M., Velickovic T. C., Valluzzi R. L., Romano A. Tolerability of imipenem in children with IgE-mediated hypersensitivity to penicillins. *J. Allergy Clin.Immunol.*, 2009;124(1):167-9.

[35] Chang C. Y., Schiano T. D. Review article: drug hepatotoxicity. *Aliment Pharmacol.Ther.,* 2007;25(10):1135-51.

[36] de Abajo F.J., Montero D., Madurga M., Garcia Rodriguez L. A. Acute and clinically relevant drug-induced liver injury: a population based case-control study. *Br. J.Clin.Pharmacol.,* 2004;58(1):71-80.

[37] Hussaini S. H., O'Brien C. S., Despott E. J., Dalton H. R. Antibiotic therapy: a major cause of drug-induced jaundice in southwest England. *Eur. J.Gastroenterol.Hepatol.*, 2007;19(1):15-20.

[38] Andrade R. J., Lucena M. I., Fernandez M. C., Pelaez G., Pachkoria K., Garcia-Ruiz E. et al. Drug-induced liver injury: an analysis of 461 incidences submitted to the Spanish registry over a 10-year period. *Gastroenterology,* 2005;129(2):512-21.

[39] Sgro C., Clinard F., Ouazir K., Chanay H., Allard C., Guilleminet C. et al. Incidence of drug-induced hepatic injuries: a French population-based study. *Hepatology,* 2002;36(2):451-5.

[40] Aithal P. G., Day C. P. The natural history of histologically proved drug induced liver disease. *Gut,* 1999;44(5):731-5.

[41] Garcia Rodriguez L. A., Stricker B. H., Zimmerman H. J. Risk of acute liver injury associated with the combination of amoxicillin and clavulanic acid. *Arch. Intern. Med.,* 1996;156(12):1327-32.

[42] Mrvos R., Pummer T. L., Krenzelok E. P. Amoxicillin renal toxicity: how often does it occur? *Pediatric emergency care*, 2013;29(5):641-3. doi:10.1097/PEC.0b013e31828e9e78.

[43] Rettie A. E., Korzekwa K. R., Kunze K. L., Lawrence R. F., Eddy A. C., Aoyama T. et al. Hydroxylation of warfarin by human cDNA-expressed cytochrome P-450: a role for P-4502C9 in the etiology of (S)-warfarin-drug interactions. *Chem. Res.Toxicol.,* 1992;5(1):54-9.

[44] Conly J., Stein K. Reduction of vitamin K2 concentrations in human liver associated with the use of broad spectrum antimicrobials. *Clin. Invest. Med.,* 1994;17(6):531-9.

[45] Korzeniowski O. M. Antibacterial agents in pregnancy. *Infect. Dis.Clin. North Am.*, 1995;9(3):639-51.

[46] Reisner S. H., Eisenberg N. H., Stahl B., Hauser G. J. Maternal medications and breast-feeding. *Developmental pharmacology and therapeutics,* 1983;6(5):285-304.

[47] Kafetzis D. A., Siafas C. A., Georgakopoulos P. A., Papadatos C. J. Passage of cephalosporins and amoxicillin into the breast milk. *ActapaediatricaScandinavica,* 1981;70(3):285-8.

[48] Pichichero M. E. Otitis media. *Pediatr.Clin. North Am.,* 2013;60(2):391-407. doi:10.1016/j.pcl.2012.12.007.

[49] Llor C., Arranz J., Morros R., Garcia-Sangenis A., Pera H., Llobera J. et al. Efficacy of high doses of oral penicillin versus amoxicillin in the treatment of adults with non-severe pneumonia attended in the community: study protocol for a randomised controlled trial. *BMC family practice*, 2013;14(1):50. doi:10.1186/1471-2296-14-50.

[50] Perez-Trallero E., Martin-Herrero J. E., Mazon A., Garcia-Delafuente C., Robles P., Iriarte V. et al. Antimicrobial resistance among respiratory pathogens in Spain: latest data and changes over 11 years (1996-1997 to 2006-2007). *Antimicrob. Agents Chemother.,* 2010;54(7):2953-9. doi:10.1128/AAC.01548-09.

[51] Iroh Tam P. Y. Approach to common bacterial infections: community-acquired pneumonia. *Pediatr.Clin. North Am.,* 2013;60(2):437-53. doi:10.1016/j.pcl.2012.12.009.

[52] Bradley J. S., Byington C. L., Shah S. S., Alverson B., Carter E. R., Harrison C. et al. The management of community-acquired pneumonia in infants and children older than 3 months of age: clinical practice guidelines by the Pediatric Infectious Diseases Society and the Infectious Diseases Society of America. *Clin. Infect. Dis.*, 2011;53(7):e25-76. doi:10.1093/cid/cir531.

[53] Woodhead M., Blasi F., Ewig S., Garau J., Huchon G., Ieven M. et al. Guidelines for the management of adult lower respiratory tract infections--full version. *Clin.Microbiol.Infect.*, 2011;17 Suppl 6:E1-59. doi:10.1111/j.1469-0691.2011.03672.x.

[54] Mandell L. A., Wunderink R. G., Anzueto A., Bartlett J. G., Campbell G. D., Dean N. C. et al. Infectious Diseases Society of America/American Thoracic Society consensus guidelines on the management of community-acquired pneumonia in adults. *Clin. Infect. Dis.,* 2007;44 Suppl 2:S27-72. doi:10.1086/511159.

[55] Habib G., Hoen B., Tornos P., Thuny F., Prendergast B., Vilacosta I. et al. Guidelines on the prevention, diagnosis, and treatment of infective endocarditis (new version 2009): the Task Force on the Prevention, Diagnosis, and Treatment of Infective Endocarditis of the European Society of Cardiology (ESC). Endorsed by the European Society of Clinical Microbiology and Infectious Diseases (ESCMID) and the International Society of Chemotherapy (ISC) for Infection and Cancer. *Eur. Heart J.* 2009;30(19):2369-413. doi:ehp285 [pii], 10.1093/eurheartj/ehp285.

[56] Jahanfar S., Ng C. J., Teng C.L. Antibiotics for mastitis in breastfeeding women. *Cochrane Database Syst. Rev.,* 2013;2:CD005458. doi:10.1002/14651858.CD005458.pub3.

[57] Paterson D. L., Bonomo R. A. Extended-spectrum beta-lactamases: a clinical update. *Clin.Microbiol. Rev.,* 2005;18(4):657-86. doi:18/4/657 [pii],10.1128/CMR.18.4.657-686.2005.

[58] Knothe H., Shah P., Krcmery V., Antal M., Mitsuhashi S. Transferable resistance to cefotaxime, cefoxitin, cefamandole and cefuroxime in clinical isolates of Klebsiellapneumoniae and Serratiamarcescens. *Infection*, 1983;11(6):315-7.

[59] Poole K. Efflux-mediated multiresistance in Gram-negative bacteria. *Clin.Microbiol.Infect.,* 2004;10(1):12-26.

[60] Martinez-Martinez L., Pascual A., Hernandez-Alles S., Alvarez-Diaz D., Suarez A. I., Tran J. et al. Roles of beta-lactamases and porins in activities of carbapenems and cephalosporins against

Klebsiellapneumoniae. *Antimicrob. Agents Chemother.,* 1999;43 (7):1669-73.

[61] Chaves J., Ladona M. G., Segura C., Coira A., Reig R., Ampurdanes C. SHV-1 beta-lactamase is mainly a chromosomally encoded species-specific enzyme in Klebsiellapneumoniae. *Antimicrob. Agents Chemother.,* 2001;45(10):2856-61. doi:10.1128/AAC.45.10.2856-2861.2001.

[62] Pfeifer Y. ESBL, AmpC and carbapenemases: emergence, dissemination and diagnostics of beta-lactamase-producing Gram-negative pathogens. *Laboratoriumsmedizin,* 2010;34(4):205-15. doi:Doi 10.1515/Jlm2010.042.

[63] Mattner F., Bange F. C., Meyer E., Seifert H., Wichelhaus T. A., Chaberny I. F. Preventing the spread of multidrug-resistant gram-negative pathogens: recommendations of an expert panel of the german society for hygiene and microbiology. *Dtsch.Arztebl. Int.,* 2012;109(3):39-45. doi:10.3238/arztebl.2012.0039.

[64] Mutters N. T., Brooke R. J., Frank U., Heeg K. Low risk of apparent transmission of vancomycin-resistant Enterococci from bacteraemic patients to hospitalized contacts. *Am. J. Infect.Control.,* 2013. doi:10.1016/j.ajic.2012.11.019.

Index

A

B

C

D

E

Q

R